THE THORAX

An Integrated Approach

DIANE LEE BSR (Honours), FCAMT

White Rock, British Columbia, Canada

ISBN 0-9732363-0-2

For my mom –
I will always remember for both of us

For my dad and my brother –
unconditional love

PREFACE, 1ST EDITION

In the literature pertaining to back pain, the musculoskeletal components of the thorax have received little attention. The reference list at the end of this text reflects the paucity of research available for review. And yet, clinicians are presented daily with the challenge of treating both acute and chronic thoracic pain. It was this challenge which initiated the clinical work presented in this text.

A biomechanical approach to treatment of the thorax requires an understanding of its normal behaviour. Without a working model, the clinician is limited to using unreliable symptoms for direction and treatment planning. If the optimal behavior of the thorax is understood, then this knowledge can be applied to the examination of the painful thorax. A systematic examination of mobility/stability of the associated bones and joints can then be done. Since function is related to structure, an understanding of the anatomy is required.

The clinical investigation began in 1990 when Jan Lowcock presented a paper on stability testing of the thorax to the Canadian Orthopaedic Manipulative Physiotherapists. I am indebted to her, and many others, for the subsequent academic and clinical discussions which lead to the evolution of the biomechanical model presented here. Much of this material remains empirical and requires validation through research.

The first chapter reviews the anatomy of the thorax as it pertains to the biomechanical model. The emphasis has been placed on osseous and articular anatomy although the muscular and neural contribution to function is acknowledged. Chapter two describes the biomechanical model and chapters three to five the clinical application of this model to examination and treatment of the thorax. The purpose of this text is to provide the clinician with the ability to assess and treat articular dysfunction of the thorax. The reader is referred to other texts for a review of postural analysis, myofascial syndromes and neural dysfunction.

I would like to extend my gratitude and recognition to Mr. Frank Crymble who was responsible for the cover design and all of the art work and photographs in this text. To my colleagues at DOPC for their ongoing support and constructive reviews of 'yet another presentation on the thorax', my special thanks. And finally, to Thomas, Michael and Chelsea, thank you.

British Columbia, 1994 D.L.

PREFACE & ACKNOWLEDGEMENTS, 2ND EDITION

It's been nine years since the first edition of this text was published and while there is still a paucity of research in the thoracic spine, there have been some significant clinical developments that warrant another look at this topic. For the most part, the biomechanical model has been accepted as written and incorporated into several schools of manual therapy instruction. The most significant change is perhaps the long held view that a restriction of articular motion implies that the joint is at fault. This change has come from a clearer understanding of what can affect the neutral zone of motion and the development of an integrated model of function which considers the role of both the mind and body on human performance. This model was developed in conjunction with Dr. Andry Vleeming (Lee & Vleeming 1998, 2002) and has been applied to the thorax in this edition, the principles of this model are described in Chapter 2. Chapter 3, biomechanics of the thorax, has been updated to include research since the first edition was published.

Chapter 4 has been updated with video clips on a CDROM to demonstrate the active and passive mobility and stability techniques previously described in the first edition. In addition, new techniques are presented which analyse the force closure mechanism (dynamic stability) of a thoracic segment. The classification of dysfunction within the thorax has been changed to follow the integrated model of function. Chapter 6 has been updated with video clips on a CDROM to demonstrate the passive and active mobilization and manipulation techniques for the thorax.

Chapter 7 is brand new for this edition and contains vital information for an exercise program aimed at stabilization of the thorax. Some of the exercises are illustrated via still photos while others can be seen on the CDROM. The information is still empirical since research is lacking in this area and comes primarily from clinical experience. This chapter reviews some of the concepts of load transfer through the body, the anatomy and function of the lumbopelvic core (Lee D G, 1999) and the application of this protocol for stabilization of the thorax. Chapter 7 is written by Linda-Joy Lee (BScPT, FCAMT) and demonstrates her phenomenal ability to integrate concepts from many models. She is a superb clinician, excited by clinical and educational challenges and I thank her for taking on this one.

A project such as this does not come together through individual effort and I would like to acknowledge the production team whose ideas and guidance have resulted in an educational product that goes beyond my original intent. Edi Osghian from DV Media Inc. co-ordinated the project and was instrumental in putting it all together, thank you Edi and yes you were right – a make-up artist was a great idea! The still photos were taken by a superb photographer, Goran Basaric whose attention to detail and lighting drove us crazy for two days but in the end – I was impressed with what a little bit of light in the right place could do! Steve Sara filmed the video clips with a camera that was almost as big as he was. No rewinds or reviews were possible – "trust me, I got it right" – and he did. And none of the photos or video clips would have been possible without the assistance of our model, Melanie Coffey, Thanks Mel for saying "Sure, I can do that." Little did she know all that we would expect from her. I have collaborated on several projects with artist Frank Crymble; and once again he came to my rescue redrawing the complicated, combined biomechanics of the thorax meeting my demands for visual simplicity, yet accuracy. His patience for my persistence has always impressed me, thank you Frank. And last, but certainly not least, thank you to Laura Galloway for designing the layout for all of this material in such a visually pleasing and easy to read format.

There are many people who have contributed to my educational and personal growth that has ultimately allowed me to give this material to you, the clinician. I would like to acknowledge my heartfelt appreciation to Dr. Andry Vleeming, who challenged me to let go of my biases and see the human experience from a different perspective and to Karen Angelucci, who taught me to explore a different way of living in my own body through exercise in the method of Pilates. As always, I am especially grateful for my family, Tom, Michael and Chelsea who allow me the time, and provide the encouragement, so necessary to continue along this path of enquiry.

British Columbia, 2003 D.L.

CONTENTS

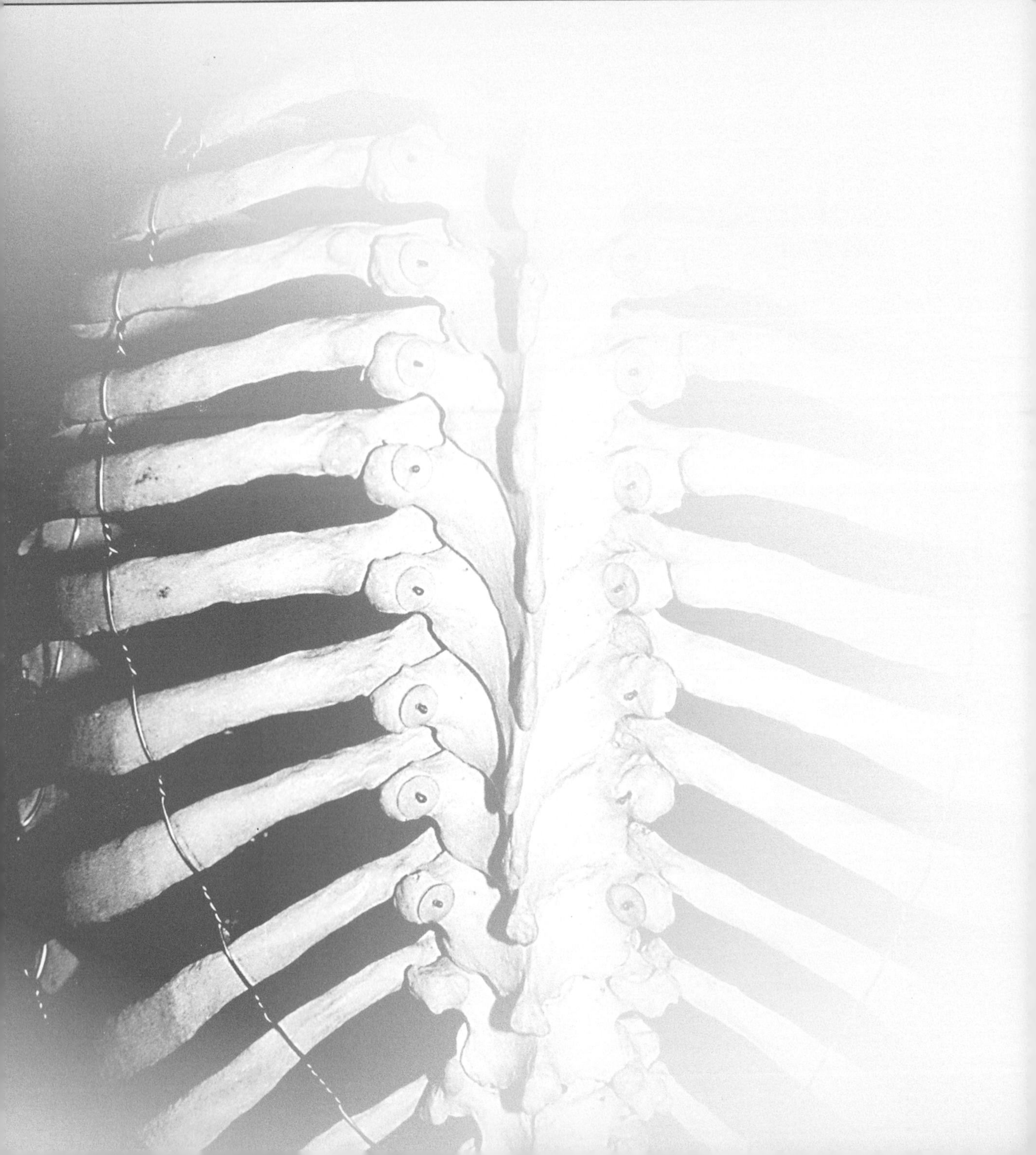

I

ANATOMY OF THE THORAX

A biomechanical approach to treatment of the thorax requires an understanding of its normal behavior. Without a working model, the clinician is limited to using unreliable symptoms for direction and treatment planning. If the optimal behavior of the thorax is understood, then this knowledge can be applied to the examination of the painful thorax. A systematic examination of mobility-stability of the associated bones and joints can then be done. Since function is related to structure, an understanding of the anatomy is required.

INTRODUCTION

The thorax can be divided into four regions (Fig. 1.1) according to anatomical and biomechanical differences. The vertebromanubrial region (upper thorax) includes the first two thoracic vertebrae, ribs one and two and the manubrium. The vertebrosternal region (middle thorax) includes T3 to T7, the third to seventh ribs and the sternum. T8, T9 and T10 together with the eighth, ninth and tenth ribs form the vertebrochondral region (middle/lower thorax). The lowest region is the thoracolumbar region which includes the T11 and T12 vertebrae and the eleventh and twelfth ribs. The regional anatomy pertinent to the biomechanical model will be described in this chapter and comes from the following sources – Gray's Anatomy (37th edition), Clinical Anatomy of the Lumbar Spine and Sacrum by Nikolai Bogduk, Clinical Anatomy and Management of Thoracic Spine Pain (eds. LGF Giles and KP Singer) and Primal Pictures 3D Interactive Series.

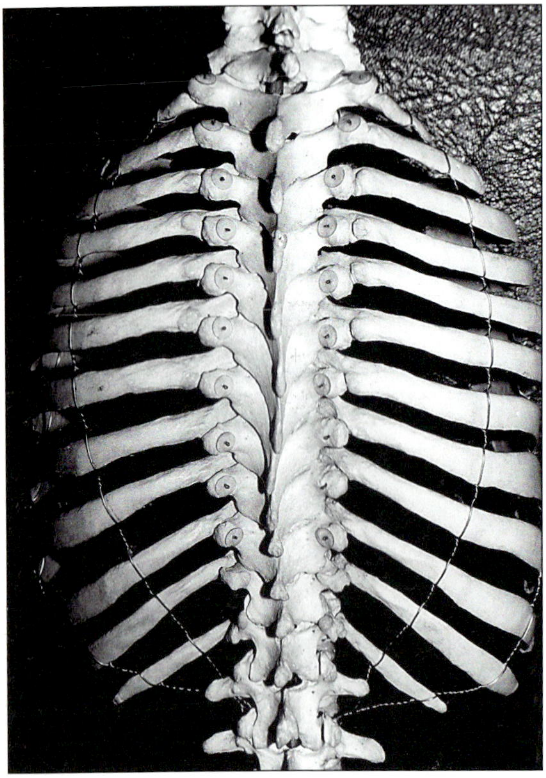

Figure 1.1. Four regions of the thorax – vertebromanubrial, vertebrosternal, vertebrochondral and thoracolumbar.

OSTEOLOGY

Vertebromanubrial Region

The first thoracic vertebra is atypical (Figs. 1.2, 1.3. 1.4). It has a large, nonbifid spinous process, clublike at its end. The superior aspect of the spinous process tends to lie in the same transverse plane as the T1-2 zygapophyseal joints. The facets on the superior articular processes lie in the coronal body plane while those on the inferior articular process present a gentle curve in both the transverse and sagittal planes. The transverse processes are long and thick. They are located between the superior and inferior articular processes at the dorsal aspect of the pedicle and are ideally situated for palpation of intervertebral motion. On the ventral aspect of the transverse process there is a deep, concave facet which articulates with a convex facet on the first rib to form the costotransverse joint. In the normal upright posture, the orientation of this joint is anteroinferior.

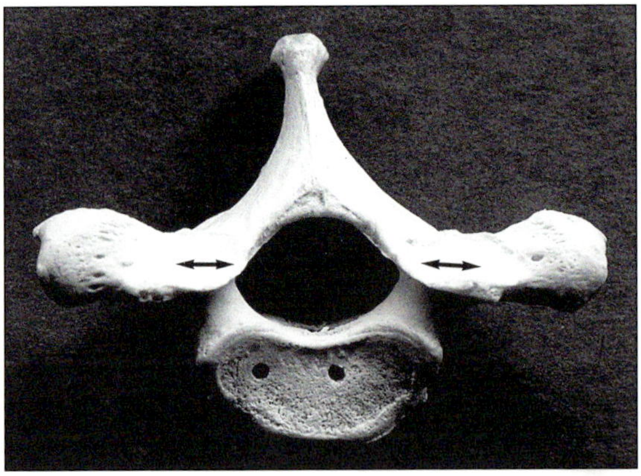

Figure 1.2. The superior aspect of the first thoracic vertebra. The zygapophyseal joints lie in the coronal plane.

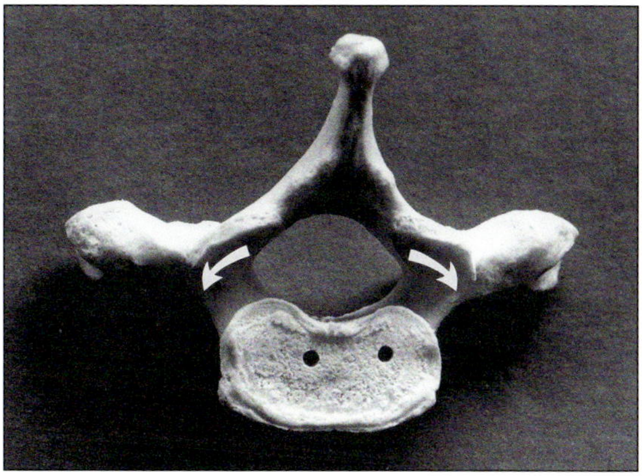

Figure 1.3. The inferior aspect of the first thoracic vertebra. The zygapophyseal joints are gently convex in both the transverse and sagittal planes. The ventral aspect of the transverse process contains a concave facet for articulation with the first rib.

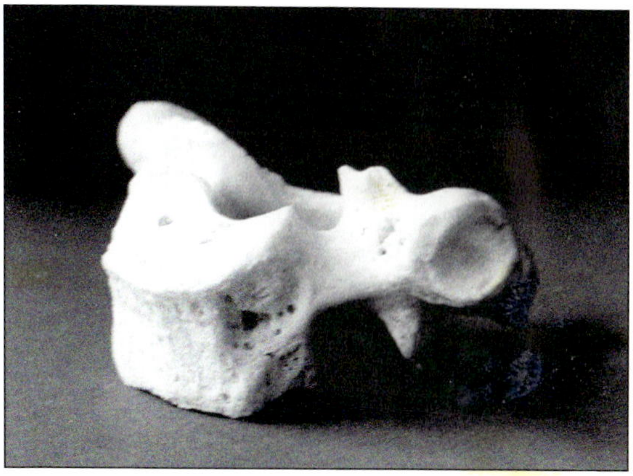

Figure 1.4. Anterolateral view of the first thoracic vertebra. The uncinate process at each posterolateral corner creates a concavity on the superior aspect of the vertebral body. There is a full facet at the superolateral aspect of the vertebral body for the head of the first rib. A demi-facet on the inferolateral aspect articulates with the head of the second rib in the second decade of life. Note the concave facet on the transverse process for articulation with the first rib.

The superior aspect of the vertebral body of T1 is concave in the coronal plane. This concavity is formed by the uncinate process at each posterolateral corner. These processes articulate with the inferior aspect of the body of C7 to form the non-synovial, uncovertebral joint (Hayashi & Yabuki 1985). There are two ovoid facets on either side of the vertebral body for articulation with the head of the first rib. The inferior aspect of the vertebral body of T1 is flat and contains a small facet at each posterolateral corner for articulation with the head of the second rib. This articulation is incomplete until early adolescence when a secondary ossification centre appears to complete the formation of the head of the rib (Penning & Wilmink 1987, Williams et al 1989). In children, the head of the second rib only articulates with T2.

The first rib (Fig. 1.5) is the shortest of the twelve and the broadest at its anterior end. The first sternochondral joint is unique in that it is fibrous rather than synovial. The first costocartilage is the shortest and this, together with the fibrous sternochondral joint, contributes to the stability of the first ring. The convex head of the first rib articulates with the body of T1 at the costovertebral joint. The neck of the rib is located between the head and the tubercle. The articular portion of the tubercle is convex and directed posterosuperiorly when the head and neck are in the

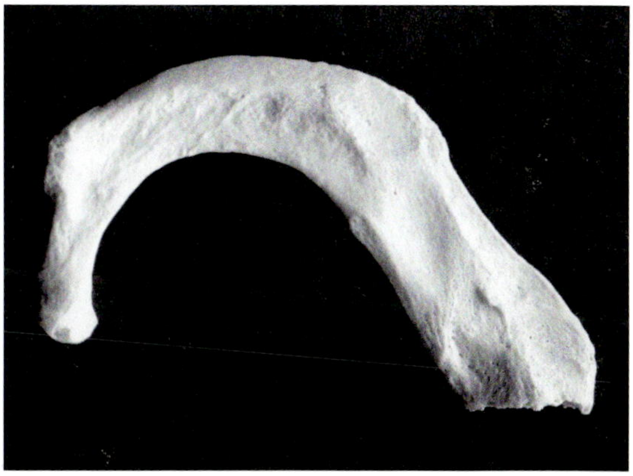

Figure 1.5. Superior aspect of the first rib.

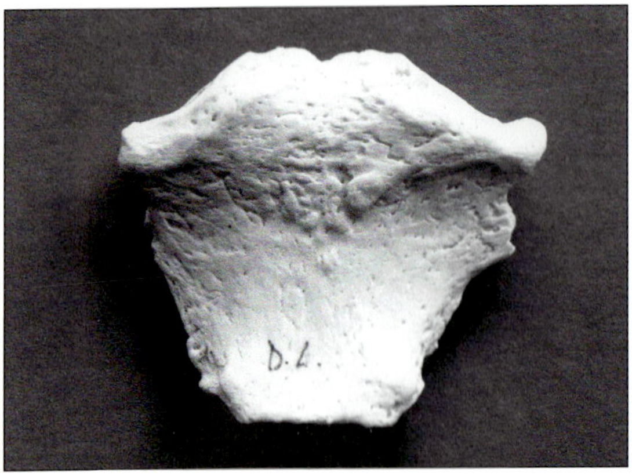

Figure 1.6. The manubrium.

normal upright posture. The second rib is about twice as long as the first and its features are similar to the vertebrosternal region described below. Anteriorly, the cartilage of the second ring articulates with both the manubrium and the sternum at the manubriosternal symphysis.

The manubrium (Fig. 1.6) is a broad triangular shaped bone which articulates with the clavicle and the costocartilage of the first and second ribs.

The manubriosternal symphysis remains separate throughout life although ossification can occur (Fig. 1.7).

Vertebrosternal Region

The vertebrae in this region (T3 to T7) have long, thin, overlapping spinous processes. The tip of the spinous process can be three finger widths inferior to the transverse process of the same vertebra and frequently deviates from the midline. Consequently, it is an unreliable point for palpating intervertebral motion.

The facets on both the superior and inferior articular processes present a gentle curve in both the transverse and sagittal planes (Davis 1959, Singer & Goh 2000) (Fig. 1.8). This orientation permits multidirectional movement. If two mixing bowls are placed one inside the other, a model of the zygapophyseal joints can be made (Fig. 1.9). The top bowl can rotate forward, backward, sideways and around the bottom bowl. Translation of the top bowl meets immediate resistance. The coronal orientation of the superior articular processes resists posteroanterior translation of the superior vertebra.

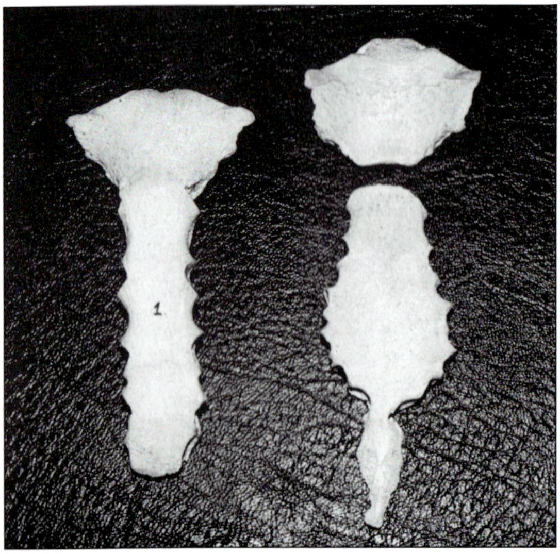

Figure 1.7. The manubriosternal symphysis is usually maintained through life, however ossification can occur.

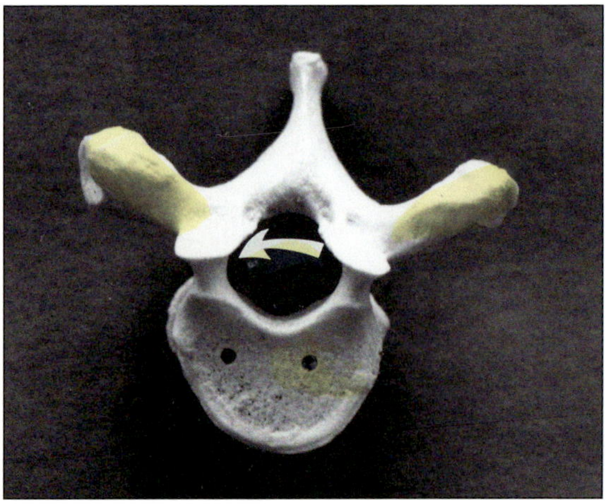

Figure 1.8. The superior aspect of the fourth thoracic vertebra. The zygapophyseal joint is gently convex in both the transverse and sagittal planes. The ventral aspect of the transverse process contains a concave facet for articulation with the fourth rib.

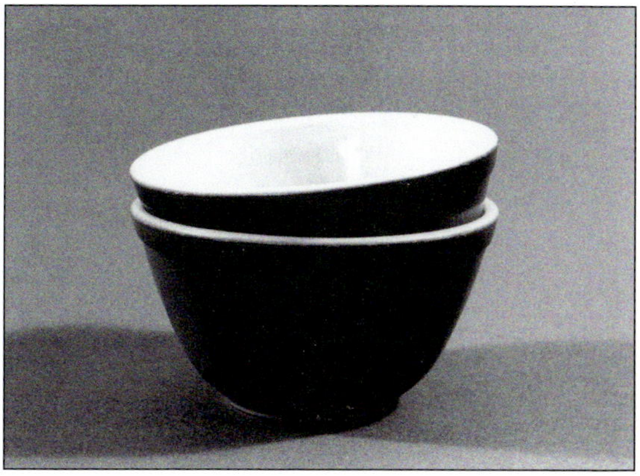

Figure 1.9. Two mixing bowls model the potential biomechanics of the zygapophyseal joints in the thorax.

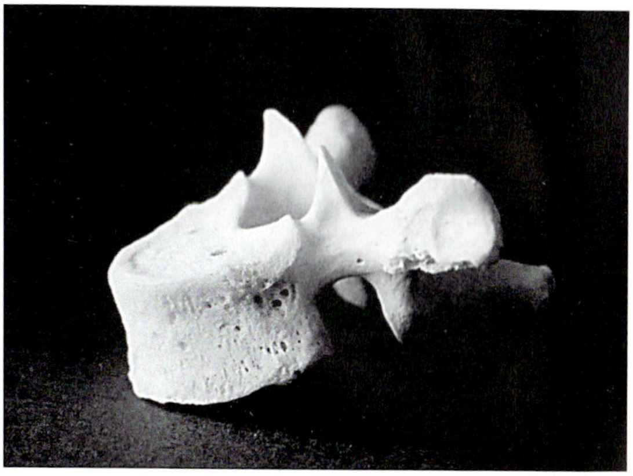

Figure 1.10. Anterolateral view of the fourth thoracic vertebra. Note the concave facet on the transverse process for articulation with the fourth rib as well as the two demi-facets on the lateral aspect of the vertebral body for articulation with the heads of the fourth and fifth ribs.

The transverse processes, located at the dorsal aspect of the pedicle between the superior and inferior articular processes, are ideally situated for palpation of intervertebral joint motion. The ventral aspect of the transverse process (Fig. 1.10) contains a deep, concave facet for articulation

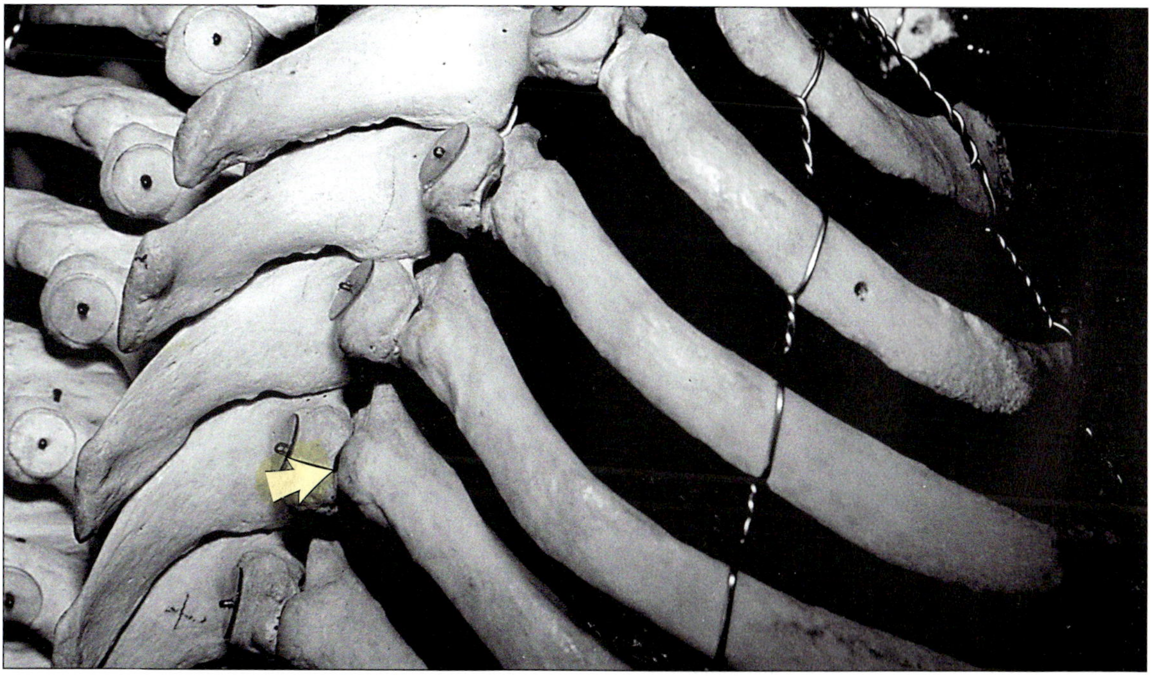

Figure 1.11. Posterolateral view of the articulated thorax, vertebrosternal region. Note the curvature of the fifth costotransverse joint (arrow).

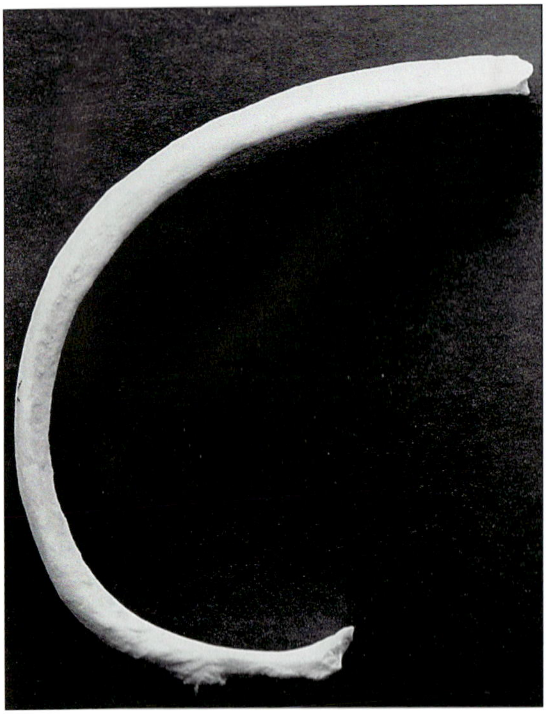

Figure 1.12. The fourth rib.

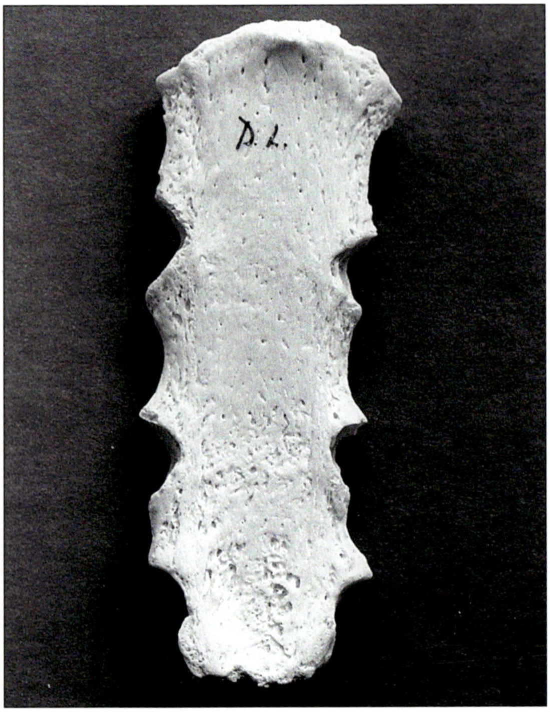

Figure 1.13. The sternum.

with the rib of the same number. This curvature (Fig. 1.11) influences the conjunct rotation that occurs when the rib glides in a superoinferior direction (see Chapter 3 – biomechanics). In the normal upright posture, the orientation of the facet on the transverse process is anterolateral.

The posterolateral corners of both the superior and inferior aspects of the vertebral body contain an ovoid demifacet for articulation with the head of the rib. Development of the superior costovertebral joint is delayed until early adolescence (Penning & Wilmink 1987, Williams et al 1989) accounting for the flexibility of the young thorax.

The shaft of the rib is long and thin and twists to a variable degree at the posterior angle (Fig. 1.12).

The sternum (Figs. 1.7, 1.13) has eight full concave facets which articulate with the costocartilages of ribs three to six. Superiorly, the second rib articulates with the sternum at a demi-facet; inferiorly, the seventh rib articulates with both the xiphoid and the sternum.

Vertebrochondral Region

The vertebrae in this region (Fig. 1.14) (T8, 9, 10) differ from the vertebrosternal region in the following aspects. The spinous process is shorter, although still directed inferiorly such that the tip lies close to the transverse plane of the transverse process of the inferior vertebra. The facet on the ventral aspect of the transverse process is flat and faces anterolateral and superior (Fig. 1.15). Therefore, when the tubercle of the rib glides superiorly, it also glides posteromedially with minimal conjunct rotation. When the tubercle of the rib glides inferiorly, it also glides anterolaterally following the plane of the costotrans-

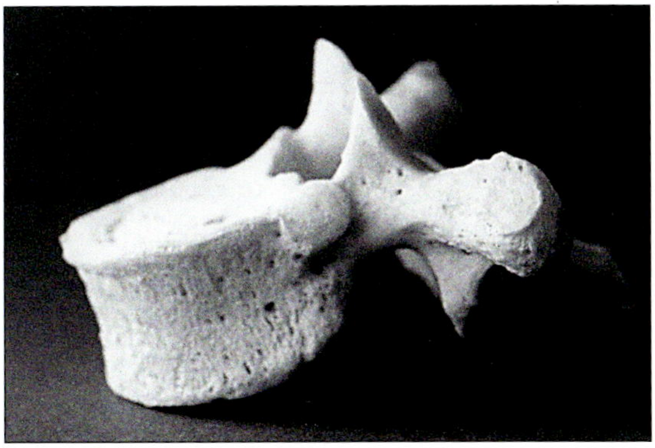

Figure 1.14. Anterolateral view of the eighth thoracic vertebra. Note the planar facet on the transverse process for articulation with the eighth rib as well as the large superior demi-facet for articulation with the head of the eighth rib and the small demi-facet for articulation with the head of the ninth rib.

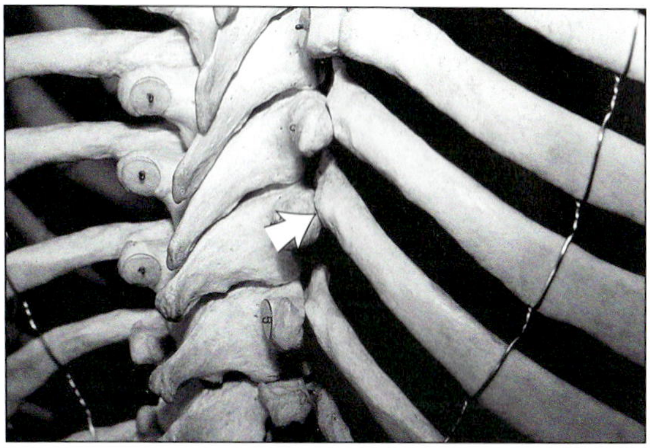

Figure 1.15. Posterolateral view of the articulated thorax, vertebrochondral region. Note the planar nature of the ninth costotransverse joint (arrow).

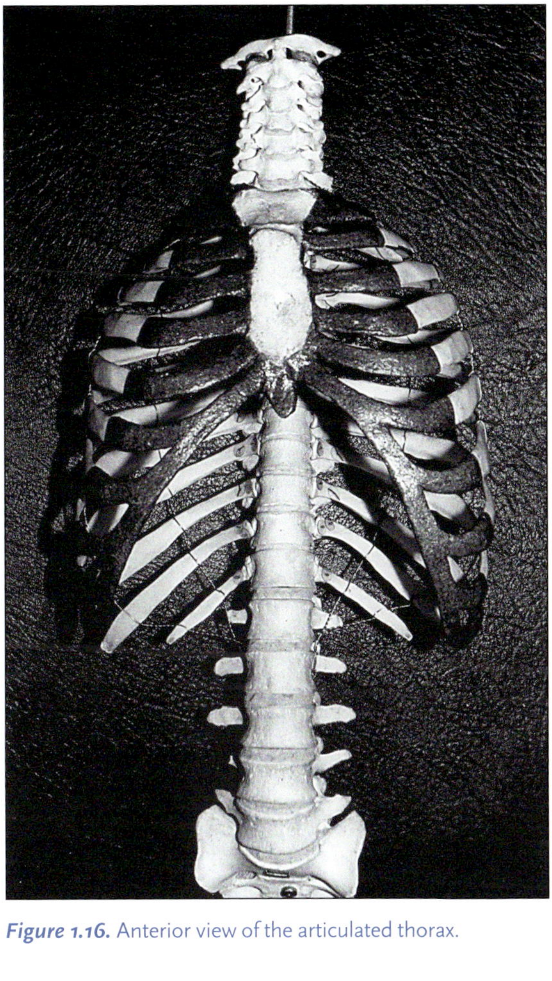

Figure 1.16. Anterior view of the articulated thorax.

verse joint (see Chapter 3 – biomechanics). The orientation of the facet for the costotransverse joint changes to accommodate greater loading from the upper limb and thorax (Giles & Singer 2000). At T2, the facet on the transverse process faces anteroinferiorly when the thorax is viewed in a normal upright posture. At T10, the facet on the transverse process faces superolaterally such that the rib rests on top of the transverse process.

T8 and T9 have four demifacets for articulation with the head of the eighth and ninth ribs. T10 is variable. Often, there is only a small articulation between the superior aspect of the head of the tenth rib and the inferior aspect of the vertebral body of T9. Occasionally, the tenth rib will articulate only with T10 at the base of the pedicle via an unmodified ovoid joint.

Anteriorly, the eighth, ninth and tenth ribs articulate indirectly with the sternum via a series of cartilaginous bars which blend with the seventh costocartilage (Fig. 1.16). There are a variable number of synovial joints between the costocartilages (interchondral joints). This arrangement permits greater flexibility.

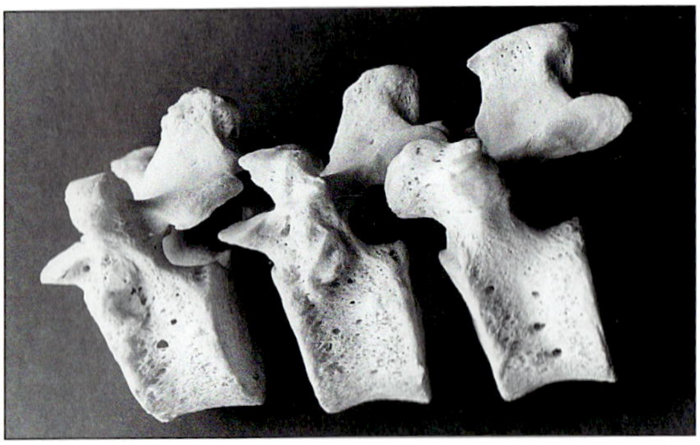

Figure 1.17. The eleventh and twelfth thoracic and the first lumbar vertebrae. Note the orientation of the zygapophyseal joints.

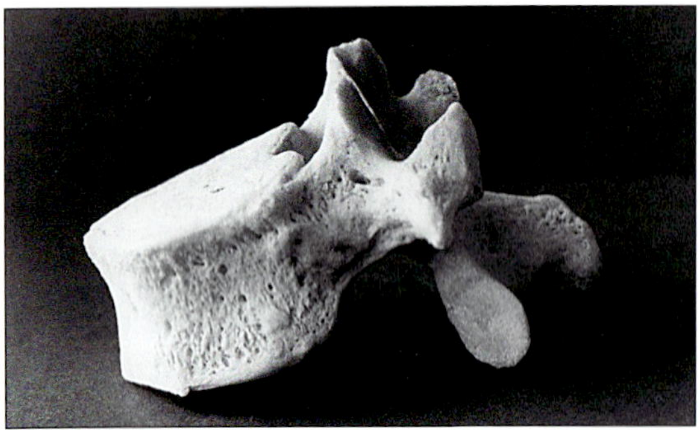

Figure 1.18. Lateral view of the twelfth thoracic vertebra. Note the change in direction of the facets on the superior and inferior articular processes. There is one facet on the lateral aspect of the vertebral body for articulation with the head of the twelfth rib. There is no facet on the small transverse process, there is no costotransverse joint.

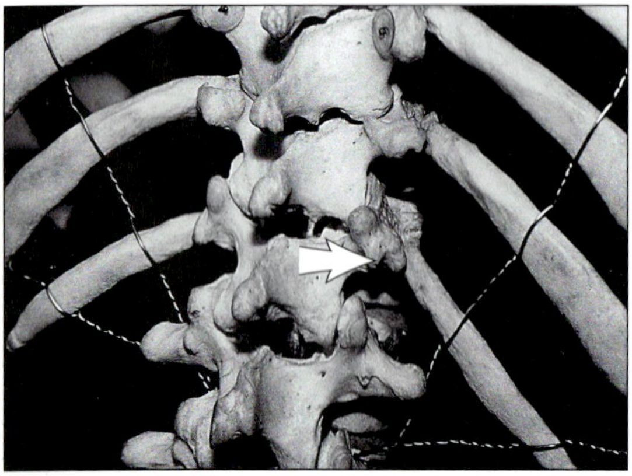

Figure 1.19. The transverse processes of the twelfth thoracic vertebrae are small tubercles (arrow) and cannot be used for palpating intervertebral motion.

Thoracolumbar Region

The spinous processes of T11 and T12 are short, stout and contained entirely within the lamina of their own vertebra (Figs. 1.17). The facets on the articular processes of T11 (Fig. 1.18) resemble those of both the vertebrosternal and vertebrochondral regions. The facets on the inferior articular process of T12 resemble the lumbar region. They have a coronal and sagittal component and when articulated with L1 restrict axial rotation. The orientation of T11-12 does not restrict axial rotation.

Laterally, the transverse processes are small tubercles (Fig. 1.19), the mamillary processes are larger and more superficial. The spinous process is a more reliable point for palpating intervertebral motion in this region.

The heads of the eleventh and twelfth ribs articulate only with the vertebral body at the base of the pedicle via an unmodified ovoid joint (Fig. 1.20). There is no costotransverse joint in this region. The ribs do not have a neck and do not twist significantly. They remain detached from the rest of the thorax anteriorly (Fig. 1.21) and provide attachment for the diaphragm and trunk musculature. The shape of the costovertebral joint facilitates multi-directional movement of the vertebral body even when the large muscles contract and fix the eleventh and twelfth ribs. The eleventh segment (T11, T12, eleventh rib) is the most flexible in the thorax.

ARTHROLOGY

Zygapophyseal Joints

The zygapophyseal joints of the thorax are synovial and, like other synovial joints, contain small intra-articular folds comprised of fibrous or fibro-fatty tissue (Giles & Singer 2000). These folds originate medially from within the joint space and extend a variable distance into the joint cavity. The capsule of the zygapophyseal joint is supported by the ligamentum flavum medially and the rotatores muscle laterally (Bogduk 1997), the deepest fibers of this muscle insert into the capsule.

Costal Joints

The costotransverse joints are synovial and also contain small intra-articular folds (Giles & Singer 2000). The lateral costotransverse ligament supports the lateral aspect of the joint and is transversely oriented (Fig. 1.22). It attaches to the tip of the transverse process and inserts into the non-articular portion of the tubercle of the rib. The superior costotransverse ligament has a variable number of bands that run in a superoinferior direction from the inferior aspect of the transverse process to the neck of the rib below. The neurovascular elements of the thoracic segment emerge between the bands of this ligament.

The second to tenth costovertebral joints are divided into two synovial cavities, each cavity is separated by an intra-articular ligament. The capsule is supported by the radiate ligament (Fig. 1.23) which has fibres extending from the head of the rib both anteriorly and posteriorly to blend with the vertebral body of the level above, the intervertebral disc and the vertebral body of the level below. The costotransverse ligament connects the neck of the rib to the ventral aspect of the adjacent transverse process. The first, eleventh and twelth costovertebral joints contain a single facet located at the base of the pedicle. They are essentially unmodified ovoid in shape.

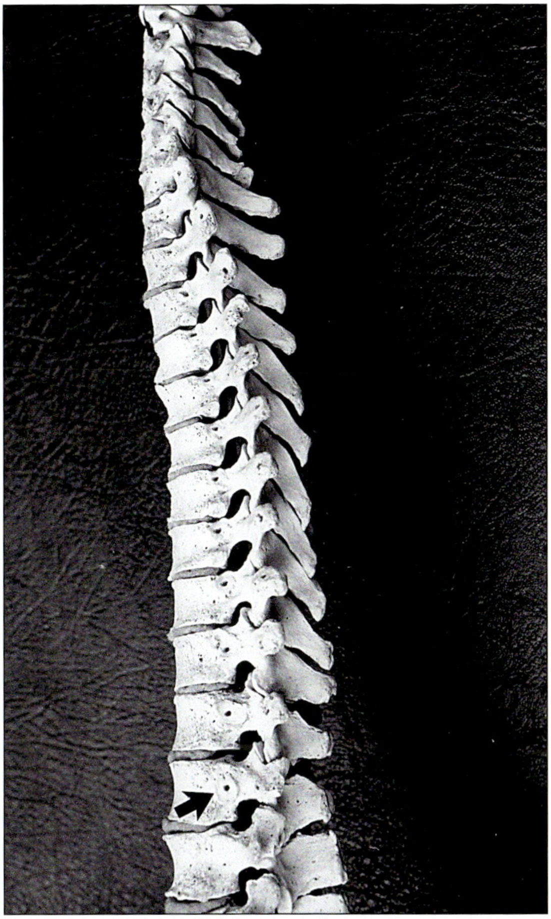

Figure 1.20. Lateral view of the thoracic spine. Note the unmodified ovoid facet (arrow) for the head of the twelfth rib.

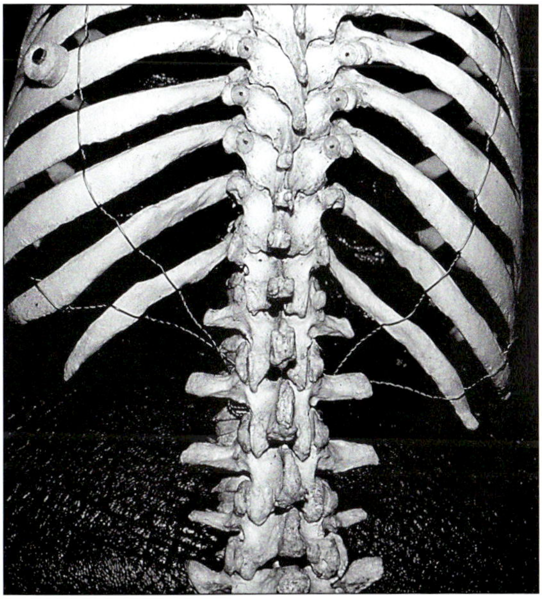

Figure 1.21. Posterior view of the articulated thorax, thoracolumbar region. Occasionally the spinous processes are bifid.

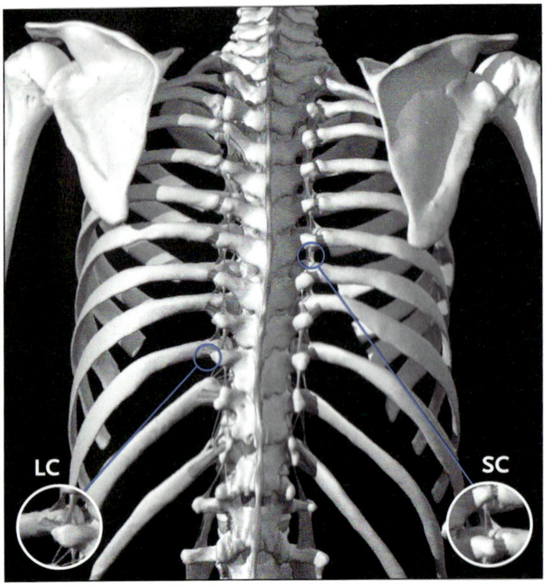

Figure 1.22. The ligaments of the posterior aspect of the thorax.
LC= lateral costotransverse ligament
SC=superior costotransverse ligament
(Reproduced with permission from Primal Pictures).

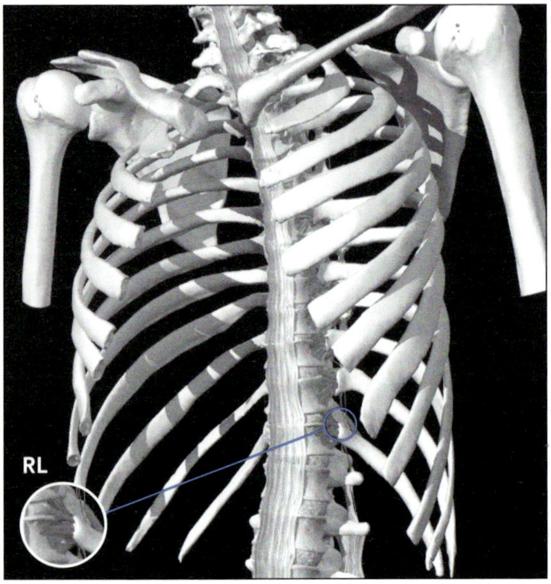

Figure 1.23. The costovertebral joint and the ligaments of the anterior aspect of the thoracic spine.
RL=radiate ligament
(Reproduced with permission from Primal Pictures).

With the exception of the first, the sternocostal joints are synovial, unlike the lateral costochondral joints which are fibrous, the periosteum and perichondrium continuous.

Intervertebral Disc

The intervertebral discs of the thoracic spine are narrower than those in the cervical and lumbar regions and constitute approximately one-sixth of the length of the thoracic vertebral column. Since the ratio of the height of the disc to the vertebral body is 1:5, motion between the segments of the thorax is small. There is a linear increase in the cross-sectional area of the disc in the lower thorax reflecting an increase in the weight bearing function of these levels.

MYOLOGY

The muscles of the thorax can be divided into deep and superficial layers. Functionally, these muscles can be classified into two systems; the local and the global (Bergmark 1989, Richardson et al 1999).

Local System – Classification

Functionally, stability is maintained via low force continuous activity of the local musculature. These muscles work in all positions of the joint and during all directions of joint motion. This activity increases the stiffness at a segmental level and helps to control excessive physiological and translational motion, especially in the neutral joint position where passive support from the ligaments and capsule is minimal. The activity of the local system often increases in anticipation of impending load or motion, thus providing joint

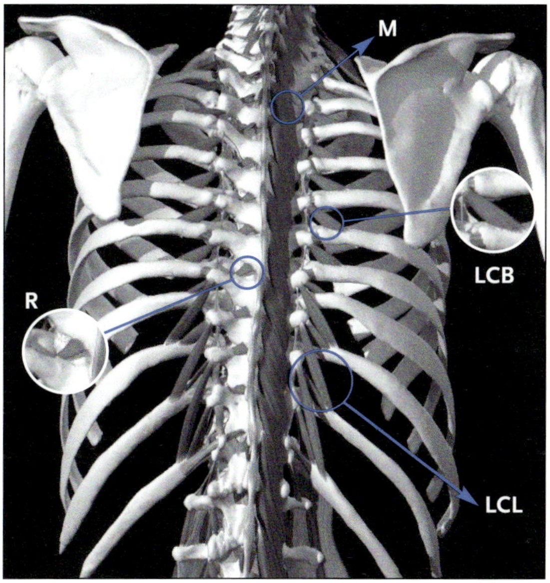

Figure 1.24. The local stabilizers of the thorax include the rotatores (R), levator costarum brevis (LCB) and longus (LCL) and the deep fibers of multifidus (M). (Reproduced with permission from Primal Pictures).

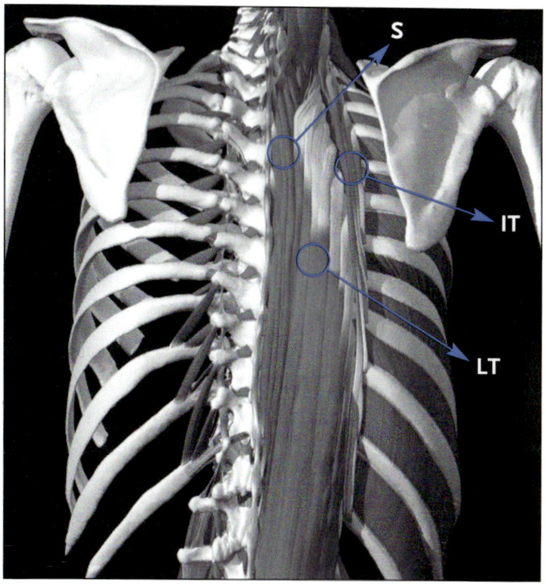

Figure 1.25. The intercostals are classified as local stabilizers while spinalus (S), longissimus thoracis (LT) and iliocostalis thoracis (IT) are global muscles. (Reproduced with permission from Primal Pictures).

protection and support (Bo & Stein 1994, Comerford & Mottram 2001, Hodges et al 1997b, Richardson et al 1999).

Global System – Classification

The primary role of the global system is to generate torque and provide control of inner and outer range of joint motion. These muscles are required to concentrically shorten into the full physiological inner range position, isometrically hold this position as well as eccentrically control or decelerate loads against gravity (Comerford & Mottram 2001, Richardson et al 1999). They are necessary for stability under conditions of high load.

In general, the deeper layers of the spinal musculature are segmental and are thought to play a significant role in local stabilization of the spine (Bergmark 1989, Hides et al, 1994 Moseley et al 2002). The superficial muscles of the thorax tend to span several segments/ribs and function to move the thorax relative to the lumbar spine and pelvis and therefore function globally. Co-activation of different muscle groups results in flexion, extension, lateral bending and axial rotation of the thorax.

Local System – Anatomy

Specifically, the local muscles which stabilize the thorax are thought to include the rotatores thoracis, the deep fibers of multifidus, the levator costarum breves and longus and the internal and external intercostal muscles. The rotatores thoracis and multifidus are part of the transversospinalis group. The research has yet to be done to confirm the inclusion of these muscles into this classification, they are here based on clinical impression and extrapolation from research done in the lumbar spine and pelvis.

The eleven pairs of rotatores thoracis (Fig. 1.24) arise from the inferior border and lateral surface of the lamina of the thoracic vertebra and run inferolaterally to insert onto the superoposterior

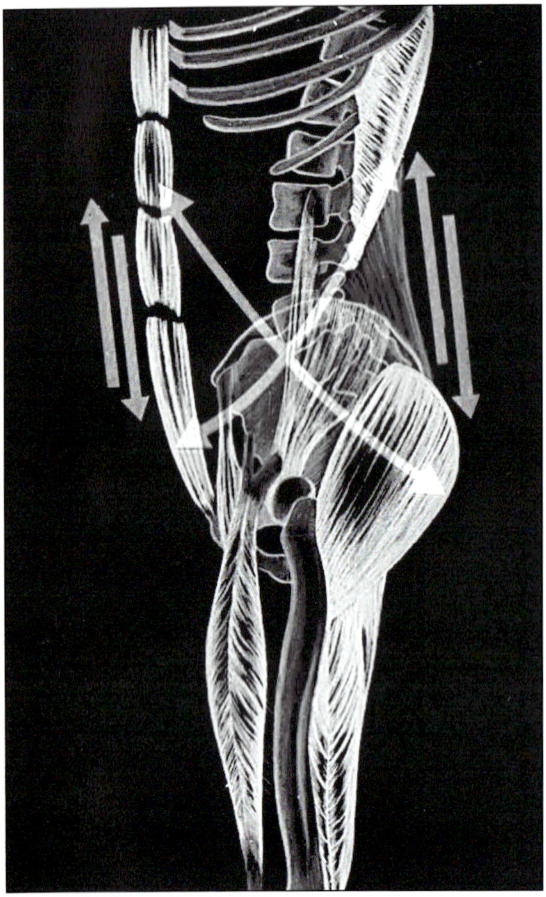

Figure 1.26. The global stabilizers and mobilizers of the thorax connect the thorax to the pelvic girdle and function to control sagittal and transverse plane motion. (Reproduced with permission from DeRosa & Porterfield 2001.)

aspect of the base of the transverse process of the subjacent segment. These muscle fibers attach to the capsule of the zygapophyseal joint.

The multifidus muscle (Fig. 1.24) overlies the rotatores thoracis and fills the gutter between the spinous processes and the base of the transverse processes. The deepest layers arise from the lateral aspect of the spinous process and pass inferolaterally to attach to the base of the transverse process. The deep fibers are segmental whereas the more superfical fibers span two to four vertebral segments before attaching. In the lumbar spine, these superficial fibers are known (Moseley et al 2002, Richardson et al 1999) to be phasic in function (responsible for angular motion) whereas the deep fibers have a more tonic function (are non-direction specific and responsible for stabilization). The research is still lacking for the thorax – however the clinical impression is that the function is similar. All fascicles arising from the spinous process of a given vertebra are innervated by the medial branch of the dorsal ramus of that segment (Bogduk 1997) regardless of the length or depth of the muscle.

The levator costarum breves (Fig. 1.24) are found from C7 to T11 and arise from the tip of the transverse process. The short fibers pass inferolaterally to insert onto the subjacent rib between the tubercle and the angle. The levator costarum longus is comprised of four muscular slips which arise from the transverse processes of T7, T8, T9 and T10 (vertebrochondral region only). The fibers are longer than those of levator costarum breves and pass inferolaterally to insert between the tubercle and angle of the rib two segments below their origin.

The intercostal muscles (internal and external) (Fig. 1.25) fill the gap between the ribs and although their action is facilitated with expiration and inspiration respectively, their main function is to stiffen the chest wall during respiration. In this regard, they are non-direction specific thus meeting the criteria for being local stabilizers. The internal intercostal muscle lies deep to the external intercostal muscle and arises from the subcostal groove and costal cartilage and passes inferolateral anteriorly and inferomedial posteriorly. The external intercostal muscle arises from the lower border of the rib passing inferolateral posteriorly and inferomedial anteriorly until the costochondral joint beyond which it continues to attach to the sternum as the external intercostal membrane.

Global System – Anatomy

The global muscles of the thorax (Fig. 1.26) include the external and internal oblique abdominals, semispinalis thoracis, erector spinae, rectus abdominis and possibly the upper fibers of transverses abdominis. All of these muscles generate torque and function to control direction specific movements. The oblique abdominals control rotation of the thorax relative to the lumbar spine and pelvic girdle concentrically, isometrically and eccentrically.

The external oblique is the largest and most superficial abdominal with eight digitations arising from the external surfaces and inferior borders of the lower eight ribs. This origin interdigitates with fibers of serratus anterior and latissimus dorsi. The upper attachments of the external oblique arise close to the costochondral joints, the middle attachments to the body of the ribs and the lowest to the tip of the cartilage of the 12th rib. Inferiorly, the posterior fibers descend vertically to attach to the outer lip of the anterior 1/2 of the iliac crest. The upper and middle fibers end in the anterior abdominal aponeurosis (Fig. 1.27). Rizk (1980) investigated this structure in 41 specimens and discovered that the aponeurosis of the external oblique was bilaminar. The two layers cross the midline to blend with the fascia of the opposite side with the deep layer being continuous with the contralateral internal oblique. The superficial layer merges with the superficial layer of the contralateral side. The deep and superficial layers produce a cross hatched appearance as their orientation is 90° to one another.

The internal oblique lies between the external oblique and the transversus abdominis and arises from the lateral 2/3 of the inguinal ligament, anterior 2/3 of the intermediate line of the iliac crest and the lateral raphe of the thoracodorsal fascia. The posterior fibers ascend laterally to reach the tips of the 11th and 12th ribs and the 10th rib near the costochondral junction. The anterior fibers arising from the inguinal ligament arch inferomedially to blend with the aponeurosis of transversus abdominis and attach to the pubic crest. The intermediate fibers pass superomedially to insert into a bilaminar aponeurosis (Rizk 1980) blending with the aponeurosis of the external oblique forming a decussating network of fascia across the midline of the body.

Semispinalis thoracis is part of the transversospinalis group and is superficial to multifidus and deep to spinalis thoracis (part of the erector spinae group). It arises from tendinous slips from the transverse processes of T6 – T10 and inserts cranially into the lateral aspect of the spinous processes of C6-T4.

Spinalis thoracis (Fig. 1.25) (medial part of the erector spinae group) lies medial to the thoracic component of longissimus thoracis (Fig. 1.25) and posterior to the thoracic component of semispinalis. It arises from the lateral aspect of the spinous process from T11-L2. From these 4 slips it forms a small muscle which inserts cranially into the lateral aspect of the spinous process of T1-T8.

The thoracic component of longissimus thoracis (Fig. 1.25) is the largest part of the erector spinae group in the thoracic spine and forms the bulk of the paravertebral muscle mass adjacent to the spine. It arises from the ribs and transverse processes of T1 – T12 and descends to attach via the aponeurosis of the erector spinae to the spinous processes of the lumbar spine and sacrum. Each fascicle descends a variable length with those from the upper thorax reaching to L3 while the lower fascicles bridge the lumbar spine completely.

Iliocostalis thoracis (Fig. 1.25) (lateral part of the erector spinae) lies lateral to longissimus and medial to the thoracic component of iliocostalis lumborum. It arises from the superior border of

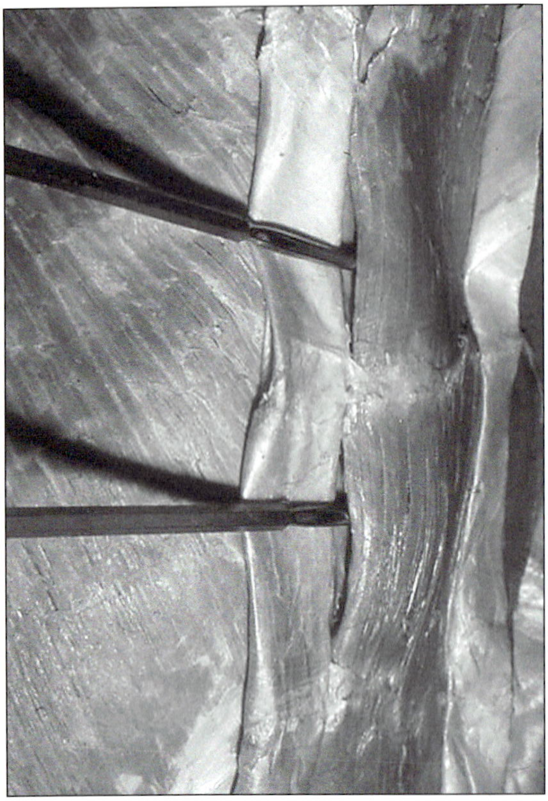

Figure 1.27. The anterior fibers of the external oblique muscle insert into the abdominal fascia strongly connecting to the interdigitations separating the rectus abdominis. (Reproduced with permission from DeRosa & Porterfield 2001).

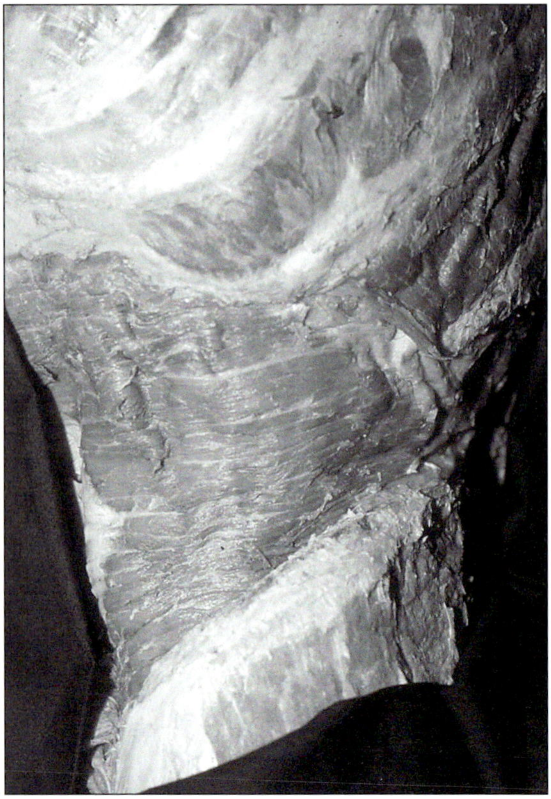

Figure 1.28. Transversus abdominis. (Reproduced with permission from DeRosa & Porterfield 2001).

the angle of ribs seven to twelve inserting into the superior border of the angle of ribs one to six and the transverse process of C7. This muscle is contained entirely within the thorax.

The thoracic component of iliocostalis lumborum (Bogduk 1997) is large and the most lateral part of the erector spinae muscle group. Fascicles from the inferior borders of the angles of the lower seven to eight ribs originate lateral to the attachment of iliocostalis thoracis and descend to attach to the ilium and sacrum with the thoracic component of the longissimus thoracis to form the aponeurosis of erector spinae. These thoracic fascicles have no attachment to the lumbar vertebra bridging the gap between the thorax and the pelvis. Since the thoracic component of iliocostalis lumborum lies lateral to the axis of spinal rotation and the distance between the rib cage and the pelvis is greatly increased during contralateral rotation, Bogduk (1997) suggests that this muscle can serve to derotate the thoracic cage and thus could also qualify as a global muscle for this region.

Rectus abdominis (Fig. 1.27) lies posterior to the anterior abdominal fascia separated from its counterpart by the linea alba. It is divided by three tendinous intersections which are connected to the external oblique laterally (DeRosa 2001). It arises from the fifth to seventh ribs and the xyphoid process and descends to attach to the pubic crest and tubercle.

Transversus abdominis (Fig. 1.28) is the deepest abdominal and arises from the lateral 1/3 of the inguinal ligament, the anterior 2/3 of the inner lip of the iliac crest, the lateral raphe of the thoracodorsal fascia and the internal aspect of the lower six costal cartilages interdigitating with the costal fibers of the diaphragm. From this broad attachment, the muscle runs transversely around the trunk where its upper and middle fibres blend with the fascial envelope of the rectus abdominis reaching the linea alba in the midline. Inferiorly, the muscle blends with the insertion of the internal oblique muscle to reach the pubic crest. The lower fibers of transversus abdominis are known (Hodges et al 1997a,b) to locally stabilize the lumbopelvic region. Urquhart et al (2001) noted that the upper and middle fibers of transverses abdominis tend to be more direction specific with respect to rotation of the thorax. It is possible that these fibers are part of the global system.

The Integrated Model of Function

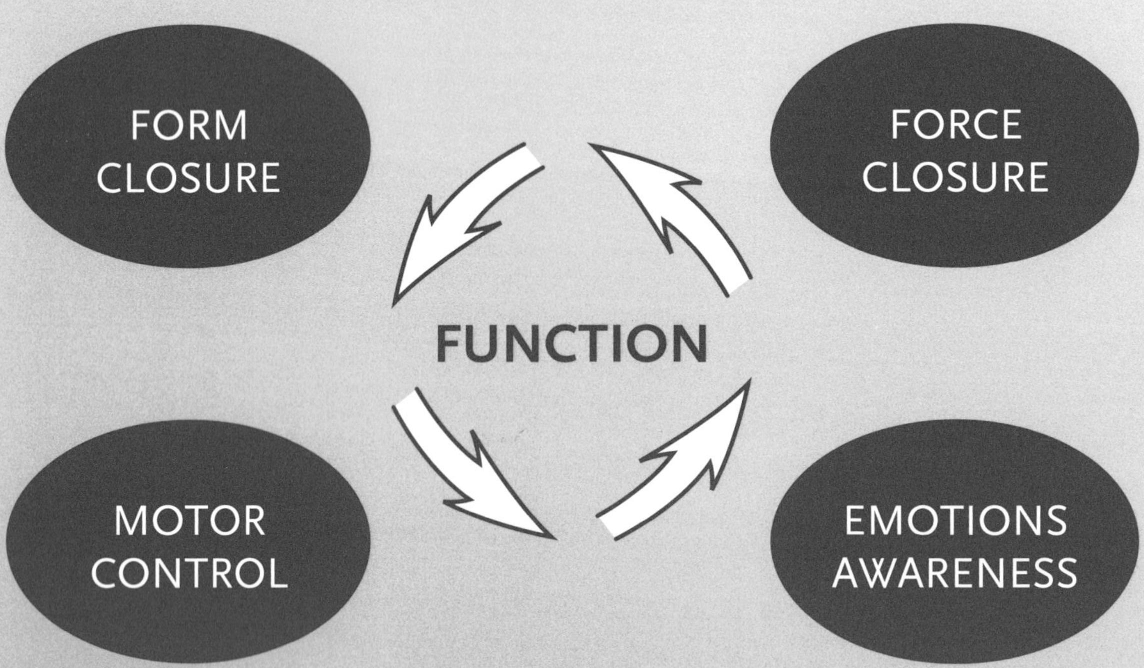

2

PRINCIPLES OF THE INTEGRATED MODEL OF FUNCTION

The following text is taken in part from material jointly written by the author and Dr. Andry Vleeming (Lee & Vleeming 2002). The integrated model of function was developed from scientific and clinical studies on the anatomy and function of the lumbopelvic region and has been adapted for the thorax by D G Lee.

INTRODUCTION

Scientific research has led to the development of models that enhance our knowledge, facilitate communication and foster a unified approach to future research. The intention of the biomechanical model presented in the first edition of this text was to focus on how the joints of the thorax behaved normally and how dysfunction could be assessed and treated to alleviate symptoms. While this model did address the articular component of the patient's problem, it has become evident that two other factors can have an equal impact on recovery. These components are neuromyofascial and emotional.

The integrated model (Fig. 2.1) has four components – three that are physical

- form closure (structure),
- force closure (forces produced by myofascial action) and
- motor control (specific timing of muscle action/inaction during loading)

and one that is psychological

- emotions.

The proposal is that joint mechanics can be influenced by multiple factors (articular, neuromuscular and emotional) and that management requires attention to all.

Living on earth requires a constant response to gravity. Our upright posture requires that the gravitational force be transferred through the thorax, low back, and pelvis to the legs. How well this load is transferred over a lifetime, dictates how efficient function will be. Impairment implies that the individual has lost the ability to perform and this loss is usually associated with symptoms significant enough to motivate them to seek help. Thoracic impairment, therefore, can be defined as an inability to perform due to problems within the thorax. This impairment may be neuromusculoskeletal in nature or due to the thoracic viscera.

According to Panjabi (1992) stability is achieved when the passive, active and control systems work together. Vleeming et al (1990a,b) believe that the passive, active and control systems produce approximation of the joint surfaces; essential if stability is to be insured. The amount of approximation required is variable and difficult to quantify since it is essentially dependent on an individual's structure (form closure) and the forces they need to control (force closure). The term "adequate" (Lee & Vleeming 1998) has been used to describe how much approximation is necessary and reflects the non-quantitative aspect of this measure. Essentially, it means "not too much" and "not too little", in other words just enough to suit the existing situation. Consequently, the ability to effectively transfer load through the thorax is dynamic and depends on:

1. optimal function of the bones, joints and ligaments (form closure or joint congruency)
2. optimal function of the muscles and fascia (force closure)
3. appropriate neural function (motor control, emotional state)

For every individual, there are many strategies available to achieve stability. These are based on

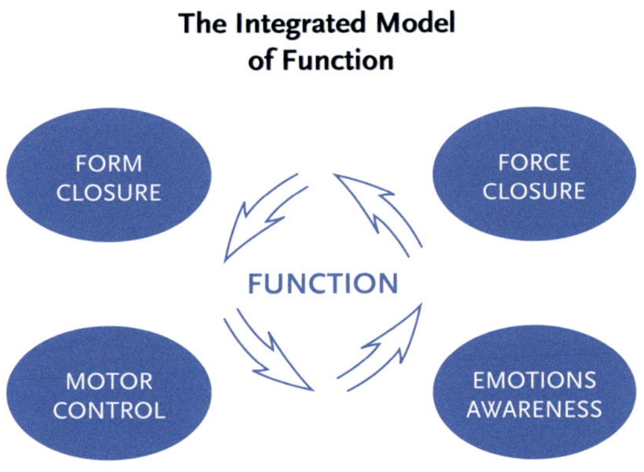

Figure 2.1. The integrated model of function – Lee & Vleeming 2002.

the individual's anatomical/biomechanical factors (i.e. connective tissue extensibility, muscle strength, body weight, joint surface shape, motor control patterns), psychosocial factors and the loads they need to control.

Stability is not only about how much a joint is moving (quantity of motion) or how resistant structures are that restrict it, but about motion control which allows load to be transferred smoothly. When motion control is inadequate, there may be too much, or too little, approximation of the joint surfaces. Too much compression over a long period of time will wear out the joints and can lead to osteoarthritis. Too little compression leads to episodes of giving way and collapse. Each component of the integrated model contributes to functional stability.

FIRST COMPONENT – FORM CLOSURE

This term was coined by Vleeming & Snijders (Vleeming et al 1990a,b, Snijders et al 1993) and is used to describe how the joint's structure, orientation and shape contribute to stability. All joints have a variable amount of form closure and the individual's inherent anatomy will dictate how much additional force is needed to ensure stabilization when loads are increased. The "form" of the thorax (the bones, joints and ligaments) has been described in detail in Chapter 1.

The thorax transfers large loads, generated primarily from the upper extremity, and its overall shape is well adapted to this task. This is mainly due to the rib cage and the effect it has on motion of the spinal segments. Andriacchi et al (1974) noted that the rib cage increased the bending stiffness of the spine by a factor of two in extension. He found that when the rib cage was left intact, the spine could support three times the load in compression before lateral instability occurred. Form closure of the thorax, therefore, depends on an intact rib cage.

There have been few in vivo studies of thoracic spinal motion and most of the biomechanics described in this text are a clinical extrapolation from Panjabi, Brand and White's in vitro investigation (1976) of the thoracic spine (see Chapter 3). This research addressed the question how much does the thoracic spinal segment move and which motions are coupled? The answer – it moves a little bit and is always coupled. Since this study was published, Willems et al (1996) investigated in vivo the direction of motion coupling and found it to be consistent for flexion/extension and variable for lateral bending and rotation. They found this to be true throughout all four regions of the thorax.

To date, no manual diagnostic tests have shown inter-tester reliability for determining how much the joints of the vertebral column and/or pelvis are moving in either symptomatic or asymptomatic subjects (Carmichael 1987, Dreyfuss et al 1994, Dreyfuss et al 1996, Herzog et al 1989, Laslett & Williams 1994). Given the wide individual variation and the limited potential range of motion, it is no wonder we have not been able to demonstrate reliability with manual testing when amplitude is considered. And yet, how can a diagnosis of hypomobility or hypermobility/instability be made without clinically reliable passive motion tests of mobility? Subsequent research has helped to clarify this dilemma.

Buyruk et al (1995a) established that the Echo Doppler could be used to measure stiffness of the SIJ. Subsequent research (Buyruk et al 1995b, 1997, 1999) using this methodology on subjects with and without pelvic pain, revealed the high degree of individual variance in the stiffness of the SIJ. Within the same subject, the asymptomatic individual demonstrated similar values for both SIJs, whereas the symptomatic individual demonstrated different stiffness values for the left and right SIJ. In other words, asymmetry of stiffness correlated with the symptomatic individual. Clinically, there appears to be a wide variation in the amount of resistance or stiffness within the thorax both between individuals of the same age and also within the same individual as a result of increasing age. In keeping with this research, the emphasis of manual motion testing should focus less on how much a joint is moving and more on the symmetry, or asymmetry of the motion palpated. A clinical reasoning approach which considers all of the findings from the examination is required to determine if the amplitude of motion is less, or more, than optimal for that individual.

Form closure analysis requires an evaluation of both the neutral zone and elastic zone of motion (Fig. 2.2) (Panjabi 1992). The neutral zone is a small range of movement near the joint's neutral position where minimal resistance is given by the osteoligamentous structures. The elastic zone is the part of the motion from the end of the neutral zone up to the joint's physiological limit.

Panjabi (1992) found that the size of the neutral zone increased with injury, articular degeneration and/or weakness of the stabilizing musculature and that this was a more sensitive indicator than angular range of motion for detecting instability. Lee & Vleeming (1998) suggest that the neutral zone is not only affected quantitatively, but also qualitatively when compression is applied (or reduced) across the joint. This compression can affect the stiffness of the neutral zone of motion. To explain this further we need to understand what compresses the thorax, in other words what provides force closure.

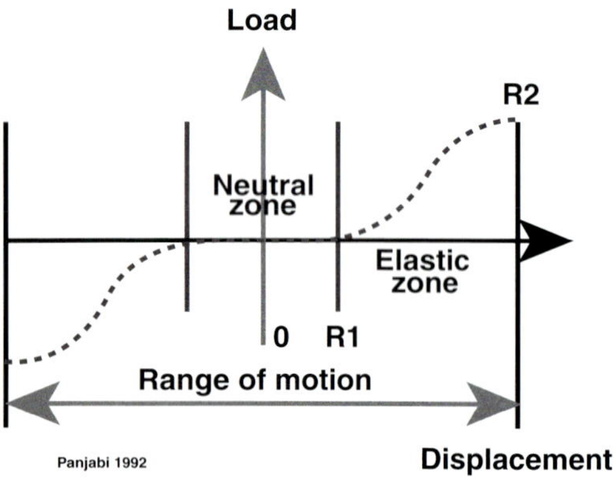

Figure 2.2. The zones of articular motion – the neutral zone (0-R1) and the elastic zone (R1-R2) (Panjabi 1992).

SECOND COMPONENT – FORCE CLOSURE

If the articular surfaces of the thorax were constantly and completely compressed, mobility would not be possible. However, compression during loading is variable and therefore motion is possible and stabilization required. This is achieved by increasing compression across the joint surface at the moment of loading – force closure (Vleeming et al 1990, Snijders et al 1993). The anatomical structures responsible for this are the ligaments, muscles and fascia. Several ligaments, muscles and fascial systems contribute to force closure of the thorax. When working efficiently, the shear forces between the vertebrae and ribs are adequately controlled and loads can be transferred between the trunk, pelvis arms and legs.

Panjabi et al (1981) tested the stability of the thoracic spinal unit by loading it to failure in both flexion and extension. Failure was defined as complete separation of the two vertebrae or more than 10 mm of translation or 45 degrees of rotation. The ligaments were then cut sequentially and the contribution of the various ligaments to stability was noted. In flexion, they found that the unit remained stable until the costovertebral joint was cut. The integrity of the posterior one-third of the disc and the costovertebral joints is critical to anterior translation stability in the thorax.

Panjabi et al (1981) then sequentially cut the anterior longitudinal ligament, the anterior half of the intervertebral disc, the costovertebral joints and the posterior half of the intervertebral disc and noted the contribution of each to stability in extension. In extension, they found that the unit remained stable until the posterior longitudinal ligament was cut. All of the ligaments anterior to and including the posterior longitudinal ligament limit extension of the thoracic spinal unit.

With respect to the neuromyofascial system, stabilization of the thorax requires both segmental (local) and global control. Segmentally, the local muscles (deep fibers of multifidus, rotatores breves, levator costarum and the intercostals) are important. Globally, the thorax is part of a larger system whose stabilization begins with the lumbopelvic core. To understand the exercise program in Chapter 7 it is essential to review how stability is achieved in the entire trunk and the research that has led to the proposals presented later in this text for stabilization of the thorax.

Lumbopelvic Stabilization – The Research Reviewed

There are two important groups of muscles that contribute to stability of the trunk. Collectively they have been called the inner unit (Richardson et al 1999) or local system (Bergmark 1989, Comerford & Mottram 2001)) and the outer unit (Richardson et al 1999) or global system (Bergmark 1989, Comerford & Mottram 2001). The local stabilizers of the lumbopelvic region consist of the muscles of the pelvic floor, the transversus abdominis, the deep fibers of multifidus, the diaphragm and possibly the posterior fibers of psoas (Gibbons 2002). The outer unit or global system consists of several slings or systems of muscles that are anatomically connected and functionally related (Meyers 2001, Vleeming et al 1995b).

The Inner Unit – Local System – The Core

The function of the local muscles is to apply adequate compression such that the system is stabilized in preparation for the addition of external loads. Research has shown (Bo & Stein 1994, Constantinou & Govan 1982, Hodges 1997b, Hodges & Gandevia 2000, Sapsford et al 2001) that the local muscle system is anticipatory when functioning optimally. In other words, these muscles work at low levels at all times and increase their action before any further loading or motion occurs.

Hodges & Richardson (1996, 1997a) have shown that transversus abdominis is an anticipatory muscle for stabilization of the low back and pelvis. Although it doesn't directly cross the SIJ, it has an impact on compression of the pelvis (Richardson et al 2002) through, in part, its direct pull on the large attachment to the middle layer and the deep lamina of the posterior layer of the thoracodorsal fascia (TDF) (Barker & Briggs 1999, Vleeming et al 1995a) (Fig. 2.3a,b). As an anticipatory muscle, it is recruited prior to the initiation of any movement of the upper or lower extremity (Hodges & Richardson 1996).

In a study of patients with chronic low back pain, a timing delay was found in which transversus abdominis failed to anticipate the initiation of arm and/or leg motion (Hodges & Richardson 1997a). Delayed activation of transversus abdominis means that the TDF is not pretensed and the pelvis is therefore not compressed in preparation for external loading. Therefore, it is potentially vulnerable to the loss of intrinsic stabilization.

Multifidus also plays a crucial role in stabilization of the pelvic girdle. This muscle is contained between the lamina of the vertebrae/dorsal aspect of the sacrum and the deep layers of the thoracodorsal fascia. When it contracts, it broadens and therefore increases the tension of the thora-

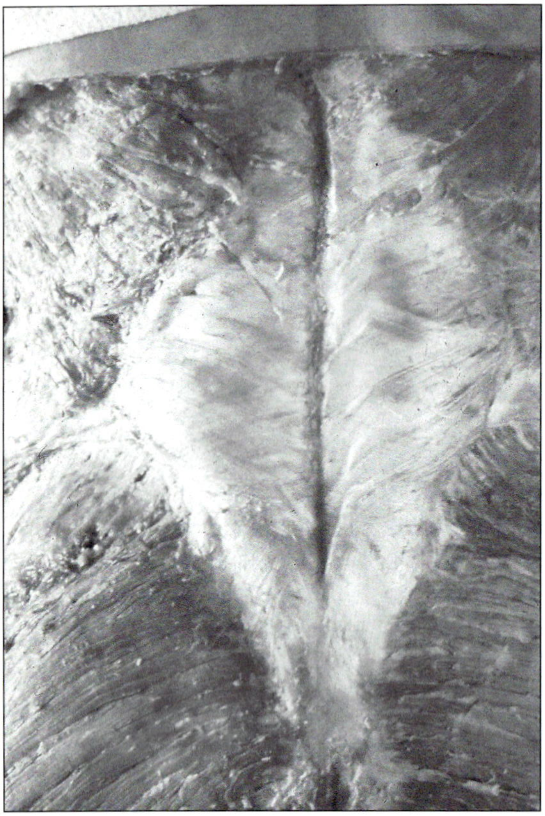

Figure 2.3a. The superficial fibers of the thoracodorsal fascia bridge the pelvis connecting the latissimus dorsi and the gluteus maximus muscles. (Reproduced with permission from Andry Vleeming).

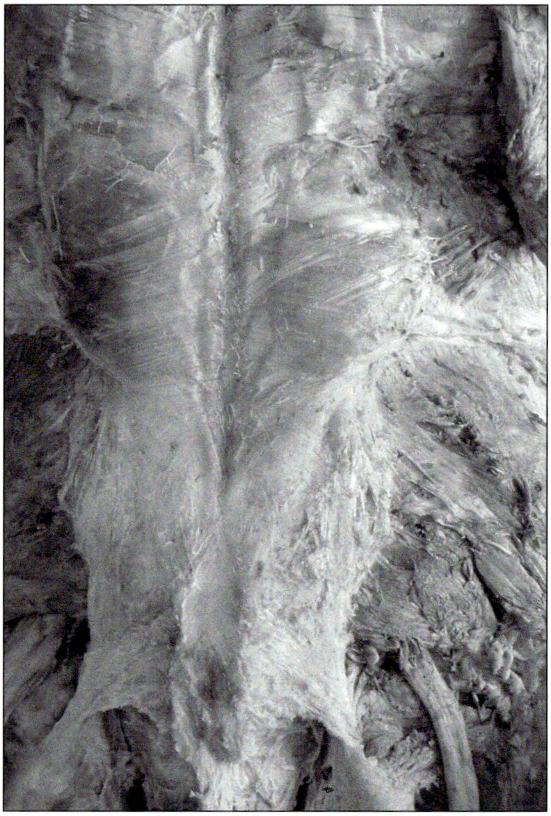

Figure 2.3b. The deep fibers of the thoracodorsal fascia form a roof over the sacral multifidus and directly connect the sacrotuberous ligament to the aponeurosis of the erector spinae muscle. (Reproduced with permission from Andry Vleeming).

codorsal fascia (Fig. 2.4a,b). This creates a "pumping up" (hydraulic amplification) (Gracovetsky 1990, Vleeming et al 1995a) effect which tenses the thoracodorsal fascia and therefore compresses the posterior pelvis (Richardson et al 2002).

The Echo Doppler has been used to measure stiffness, or compression, of the SIJ under varying conditions (Buyruk et al 1995a,b, 1997, 1999). Recently, the impact of the activation of the local muscle system on compression of the SIJ has been studied (Richardson et al 2002). The results of this research supports what is clinically noted in well trained individuals, that is – co-activation of transversus abdominis and multifidus increases the stiffness of the SIJ, facilitating the force closure mechanism of the pelvis. Further study is necessary to analyze which other muscles co-contract besides the multifidus and transversus abdominis and influence compression of the SIJ.

Hides et al (1994), O'Sullivan (2000) and Danneels et al (2000) have studied the response of multifidus in low back and pelvic pain patients and note that multifidus becomes inhibited and reduced in size in these individuals. The normal "pump-up" effect of multifidus on the TDF, and therefore its ability to compress the pelvis posteriorly, is lost when the size or function of this muscle is impaired. Rehabilitation requires both retraining

(Hides et al 1996, O'Sullivan et al 1997) and hypertrophy of the muscle (Danneels et al 2001) for the restoration of proper force closure of the lumbopelvic region. Together, multifidus and transversus abdominis form a corset of support for the lumbopelvic region. The "roof and floor" of this cannister are supported by the muscles of the pelvic floor and the respiratory diaphragm.

The muscles of the pelvic floor play a critical role in both stabilization of the pelvic girdle as well as urinary and fecal continence (Ashton-Miller et al 2001, Bo & Stein 1994, Constantinou & Govan 1982, Sapsford et al 2001). Contstantinou & Govan (1982) measured the intra-urethral and intra-bladder pressures in healthy continent women during coughing and valsalva (bearing down) and found that during a cough the intra-urethral pressure increases approximately 250ms before any pressure increase is detected in the bladder. This suggests an anticipatory reflex. The increase in urethral pressure occurred simultaneously with the increase in bladder pressure during a valsalva. They suggest the difference may be due to the role of the pelvic floor during a cough (contraction) versus a valsalva (relaxation).

Sapsford et al. (2001) investigated the co-activation pattern of the pelvic floor and the abdominals via needle EMG for the abdominals and surface EMG for the pelvic floor. They found that the abdominals contract in response to a pelvic floor contraction command and that the pelvic floor contracts in response to both a 'hollowing' and 'bracing' abdominal command. The results from this research suggest that the pelvic floor can be facilitated by co-activating the abdominals and visa versa.

When the local muscle system is functioning optimally, it applies compression to the pelvis (Richardson et al 2002) and thus stabilizes the SIJs, augmenting the form closure and helps to prevent excessive shearing of the SIJs. The pelvis is then prepared to 'accept' additional load from outside the pelvis.

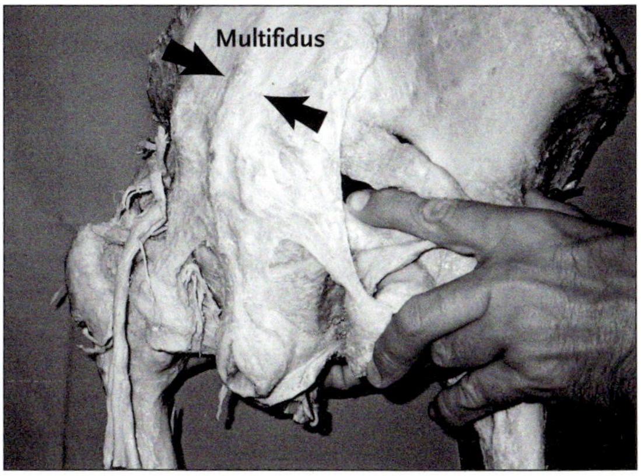

Figure 2.4a. The sacral multifidus is contained within an fibro-osseus container dorsal to the sacrum. (Reproduced with permission from Lee 2001).

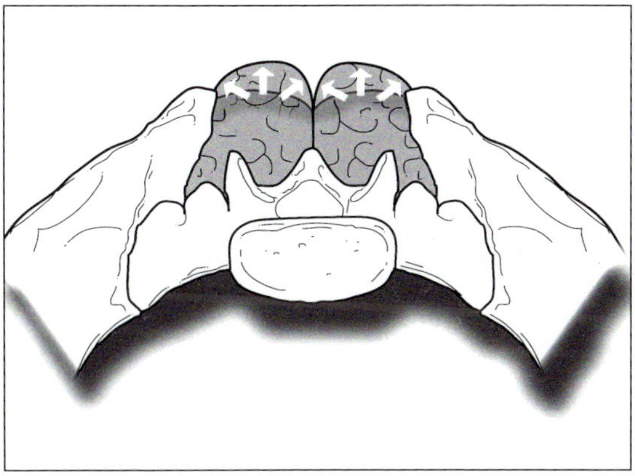

Figure 2.4b. When the sacral multifidus contracts it broadens posteriorly. (Reproduced with permission from Lee 2001).

The Outer Unit – The Global System – The Slings

In the past, four muscle systems (slings) which stabilize the pelvis regionally (between the thorax and legs) have been described (Vleeming et al 1995a,b, Snijders et al 1995). The posterior oblique sling (Fig. 2.5) contains connections between the latissimus dorsi and the gluteus maximus through the thoracodorsal fascia, the anterior oblique sling (Fig. 2.6) contains connections between the external oblique, the anterior abdominal fascia and the contralateral internal oblique and adductors of the thigh, the longitudinal sling (Fig. 2.7) connects the peroneii, the biceps femoris, sacrotuberous ligament, deep lamina of the thoracodorsal fascia and the erector spinae, and the lateral sling which contains the primary stabilizers for the hip joint namely the gluteus

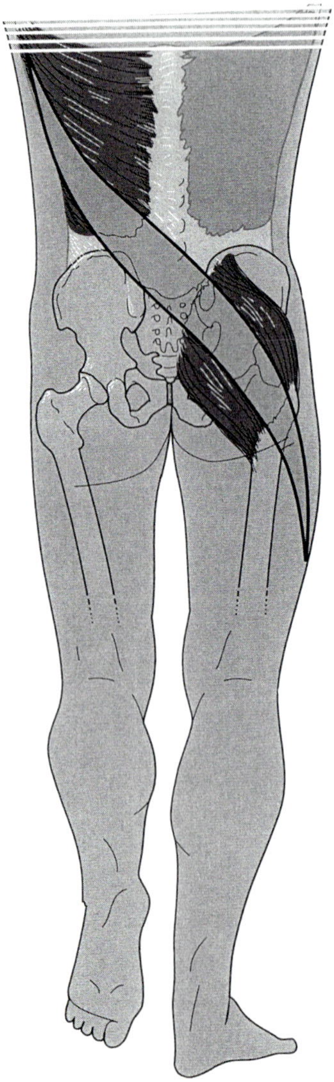

Figure 2.5. The posterior oblique sling contains, in part, the latissimus dorsi, the thoracodorsal fascia and the contralateral gluteus maximus muscles. (Reproduced with permission from Lee 1999 and Churchill Livingstone).

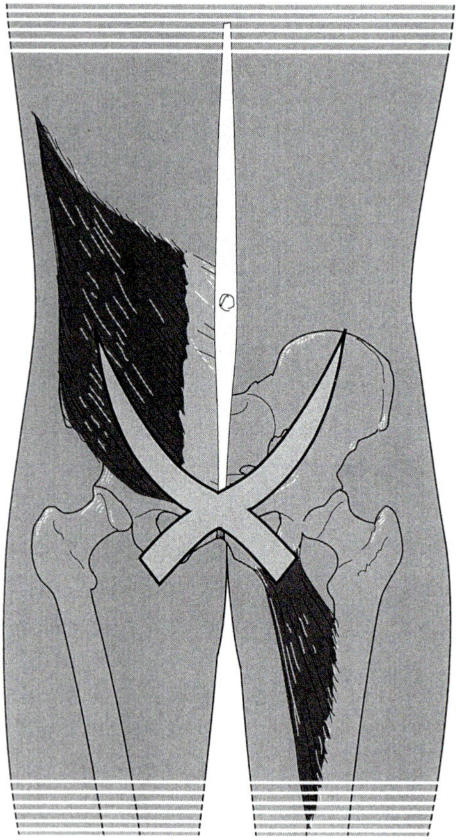

Figure 2.6. The anterior oblique sling contains, in part, the external oblique abdominal and the contralateral adductors of the thigh. (Reproduced with permission from Lee 1999 and Churchill Livingstone).

medius/minimus, tensor fascia lata and the contralateral adductors of the thigh. These muscle slings were initially classified to gain a better understanding of how local and global stability of the pelvis could be achieved by specific muscles. It is now recognized that although individual muscles are important for regional stabilization as well as for mobility, it is critical to understand how they connect and function together. A muscle contraction produces a force that spreads beyond the origin and insertion of the active muscle. This force is transmitted to other muscles, tendons, fasciae, ligaments, capsules and bones that lie both in series and in parallel to the active muscle. In this manner, forces are produced quite distant from the origin of the initial muscle contraction. These integrated muscle systems produce slings of forces that assist in the transfer of load. Van Wingerden et al (2001) used the Echo Doppler to analyze the effect of contraction of the biceps femoris, erector spinae, gluteus maximus and latissiumus dorsi on compression of the SIJ. None of these muscles directly crosses the SIJ yet each was found to effect compression (increase stiffness) of the SIJ.

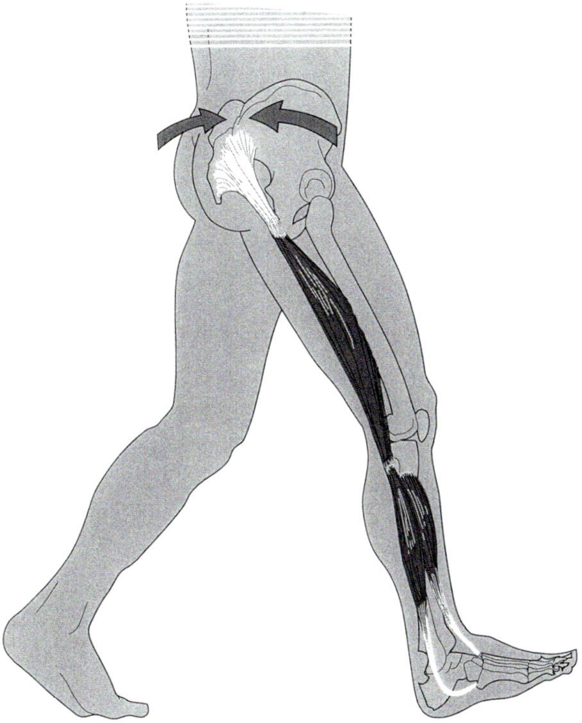

Figure 2.7. The longitudinal sling connects the peroneii, the biceps femoris, sacrotuberous ligament, deep lamina of the thoracodorsal fascia and the erector spinae. (Reproduced with permission from Lee 1999 and Churchill Livingstone).

The global system of muscles is essentially an integrated sling system which represents forces and is comprised of several muscles. A muscle may participate in more than one sling and the slings may overlap and interconnect depending on the task being demanded. The hypothesis is that the slings have no beginning or end but rather connect to assist in the transference of forces. It is possible that the slings are all part of one interconnected myofascial system and the particular sling (anterior oblique, posterior oblique, lateral, longitudinal) which is identified during any motion is merely due to the activation of selective parts of the whole sling.

The identification and treatment of a specific muscle dysfunction (weakness, inappropriate recruitment, tightness) is important when restoring global stabilization and mobility (between the thorax and pelvis or between the pelvis and legs) and for understanding why parts of a sling may be inextensible (tight) or too flexible (lacking in support).

THIRD COMPONENT – MOTOR CONTROL

Motor control pertains to patterning of muscle activation (Comerford & Mottram 2001, Danneels et al 2001, Richardson et al 1999, O'Sullivan et al 1997) in other words, the timing of specific muscle action and inaction. Efficient movement requires coordinated muscle action, such that stability is ensured while motion is controlled and not restrained. With respect to the thorax, it is the coordinated action between the local and global muscle systems that ensures stability without rigidity of posture and without episodes of collapse. Exercises that focus on sequencing muscle activation are necessary for restoring motor control (Lee 2001). The exercises in chapter 7 focus on balancing tension within the slings of muscle systems and involve an extensive use of imagery. Imagery has been shown (Yue & Cole 1992) to be effective in restoring neural patterning and increasing strength. Using imagery and specific sequencing of muscle activation, individual muscles are strengthened, lengthened and appropriately timed during functional tasks.

FOURTH COMPONENT – EMOTIONS & AWARENESS

From Andry Vleeming

Emotional states can play a significant role in human function, including the function of the neuromusculoskeletal system. Many chronic pain patients present with traumatized life experiences in addition to their functional complaints. Several of these patients adopt motor patterns indicative of defensive posturing which suggest a negative past experience. A negative emotional state leads to further stress. Stress is a normal response intended to energize our system for quick fight and flight reactions. When this response is sustained, high levels of adrenaline and cortisol remain in the system (Holstege et al 1996, Sternberg 2000) in part due to circulating stress related neuropeptides (Sapolsky et al 1997a,b) which are released in anticipation of defensive or offensive behavior.

Emotional states (fight, flight or freeze reactions) are physically expressed through muscle action and when sustained, influence basic muscle tone and patterning (Holstege et al 1996). It is important to understand the patient's emotional state since the detrimental motor pattern can often only be changed by affecting the emotional state. Sometimes, it can be as simple as restoring hope through education and awareness of the underlying mechanical problem. Other times, professional cognitive behavioral therapy is required to retrain more positive thought patterns.

A basic requirement for cognitive and physical learning is focused, or attentive, training – in other words not being absent-minded. Teaching an individual to be "mindful" or aware of what is happening in their body during times of physical and/or emotional loading can reduce sustained, unnecessary muscle tone and therefore joint compression (Murphy 1992).

CONCLUSION

It has been long recognized that physical factors impact joint motion. The model presented here suggests that joint mechanics are influenced by multiple factors, some intrinsic to the joint itself while others are produced by muscle action which in turn is influenced by the emotional state. The effective management of back pain and dysfunction requires attention to all four components – form closure, force closure, motor control and emotions with the goal being to guide patients towards a healthier way to live in their body.

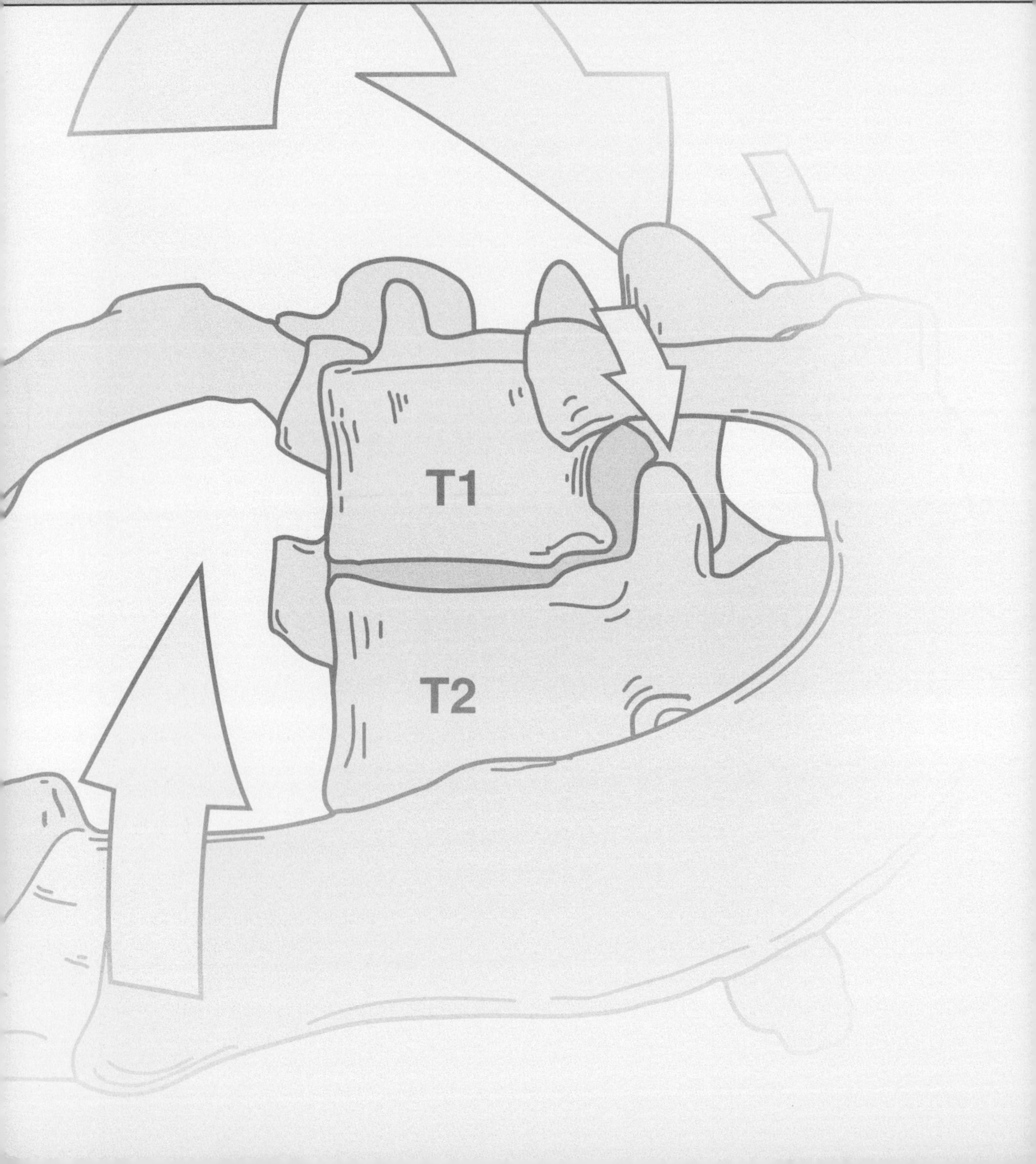

T1
T2

3

BIOMECHANICS OF THE THORAX

Managing dysfunction requires an understanding of function. The biomechanics of the thorax presented in the first edition of this text were derived from clinical observation and influenced primarily by the study of Panjabi, Brand & White (1976). Few studies have added to our knowledge base since. In 1996, Willems, Jull and Ng reported on their in vivo findings of coupled motion in the thorax. The results from this study, and the influence it has had on the original biomechanics, will be discussed in this chapter.

TERMINOLOGY

To facilitate the subsequent discussion, the terminology used requires definition. Osteokinematics (MacConaill & Basmajian 1977) refers to the study of motion of bones regardless of the motion of the joints. Angular motions are osteokinematic motions and are named according to the axis about which the bone rotates. Flexion/extension occurs about a coronal axis, anterior/posterior rotation about a paracoronal axis, sideflexion (lateral bending) about a sagittal axis and axial rotation about a vertical axis. Coupled motion refers to the combination of movements which occur as a consequence of an induced motion.

Linear, or translatoric, motions are named according to the axis along which the bone translates. Lateral translation occurs along a coronal axis, anteromedial/posterolateral translation along a paracoronal axis, traction/compression along a vertical axis, and anteroposterior translation along a sagittal axis.

Arthrokinematics (MacConaill & Basmajian 1977) refers to the study of motion of joints regardless of the motion of the bones. These movements are named according to the direction the joint surfaces glide.

LITERATURE REVIEW

Panjabi, Brand and White (1976) investigated the primary and coupled motions of the thorax in an in vitro study of several cadavers ranging in age (before death) from 19-59 years. Three hundred and ninety six load displacement curves were obtained for six degrees of motion; three translations and three rotations along and about the X, Y and Z axes (Fig. 3.1) for each of the eleven motion segments of the thoracic spine. The motion segment included the anterior interbody joint, the posterior zygapophyseal joints and the costovertebral and costotransverse joints. The ribs were cut 3 cm lateral to the costotransverse joints and the front of the chest was removed. The spinal unit was intact, however, the costal unit was not.

In 1996, Willems, Jull and Ng measured the primary and coupled motions of the thoracic spine in an in vivo study. Sixty subjects between the ages of 18 and 24 were studied using a 3 SPACE Fastrak System. The subjects were screened and excluded if they had a current or past history of thoracic pain, long term respiratory disorder or a significant scoliosis. An examination of the thoracic spine for segmental function was not done prior to the study. Sensors were attached to one spinous process in each of three regions of the thorax, one between T1-T4, a second between T4-T8 and the third between T8-T12. Each subject was seated, the pelvis and thighs secured and the lumbar spine supported. With their arms folded across their chests, each subject was asked to move to their maximal range in thoracic flexion, extension, axial rotation and lateral flexion. Each motion was carefully taught to ensure the motion

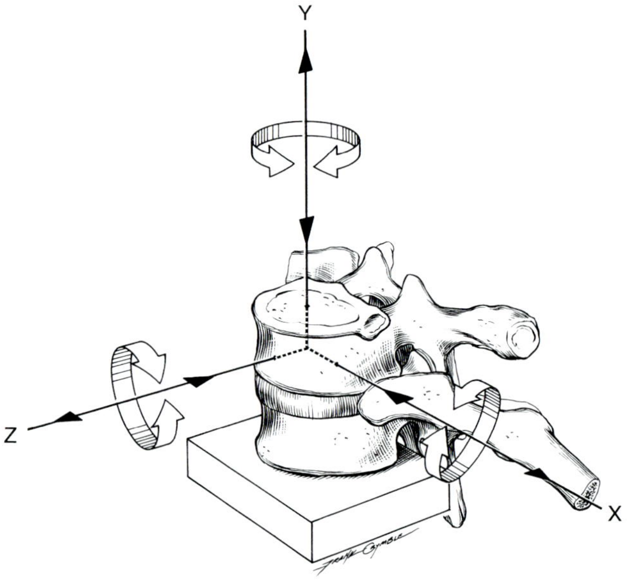

Figure 3.1 In an in vitro study by Panjabi, Brand and White (1976), 396 load displacement curves were obtained for 6 degrees of motion at each thoracic segment noting both amplitude and coupling of motion for each.

desired was actually occurring in the thorax. The Fastrak is an electromagnetic system which tracks the motion in 3D and sends the information to a computer whose software interprets the data "allowing the calculation of the position of each sensor in space" (Willems et al 1996). The methods and results from this study have been carefully considered with respect to the biomechanical model of thoracic motion and will be discussed.

According to mathematical (Samaurez 1986, Andriacchi et al 1974, Ben-Haim & Saidel 1990) and theoretical (Lee 1993, 1994) models, the thorax is capable of six degrees of motion along and about the three cardinal axes of the body; however, it is known that no movement occurs in isolation (Panjabi et al 1976, Willems et al 1996). All angular motion (rotation) is coupled with a linear motion (translation) and visa versa. As the thorax moves to meet its biomechanical demands, it must accommodate the requirements of respiration. To do this, it needs flexibility in motion patterning.

FUNCTIONAL MOVEMENTS

Vertebrosternal Region

Flexion

Flexion of the thoracic vertebrae occurs during forward bending of the trunk. Panjabi et al (1976) found that forward sagittal rotation (flexion) around the X axis coupled with anterior translation along the Z axis (.5 mm) and very slight distraction (Fig.3.2). When anterior translation along the Z axis was induced, forward sagittal rotation around the X axis and very slight compression also occurred. In the in vivo study of Willems et al (1996), sagittal plane motion was the purest and showed the least incidence of coupled motion. No axial rotation or lateral flexion should occur during sagittal plane motion of the thorax.

The osteokinematic motion of the ribs which occurs during flexion of the thoracic vertebrae was not noted in either study (Panjabi et al 1976, Willems et al 1996). Saumarez (1986) noted that

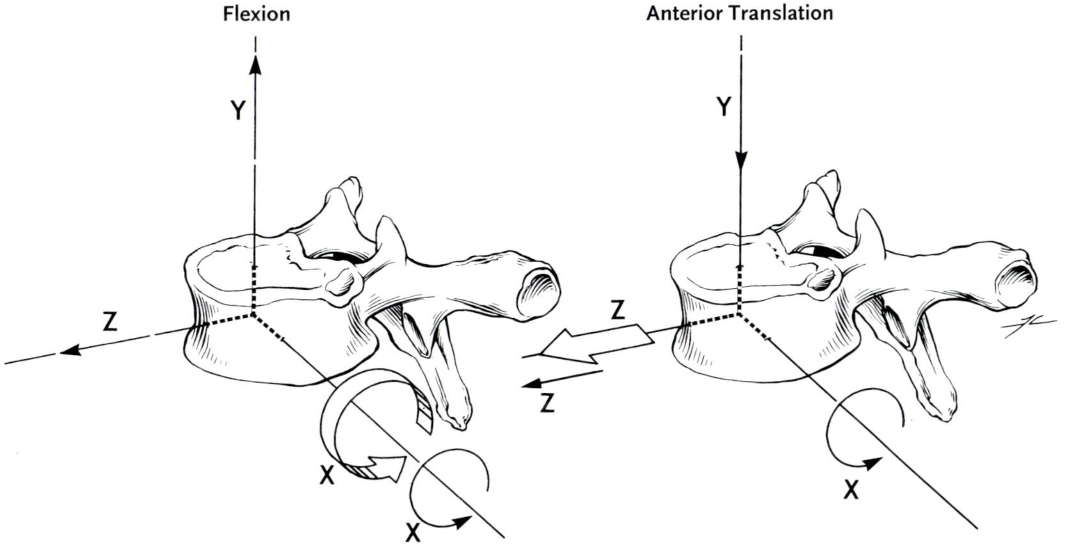

Figure 3.2. Flexion around the X axis induced anterior translation along the Z axis and slight distraction along the Y axis. Anterior translation along the Z axis induced forward sagittal rotation around the X axis and slight compression along the Y axis (Panjabi et al 1976).

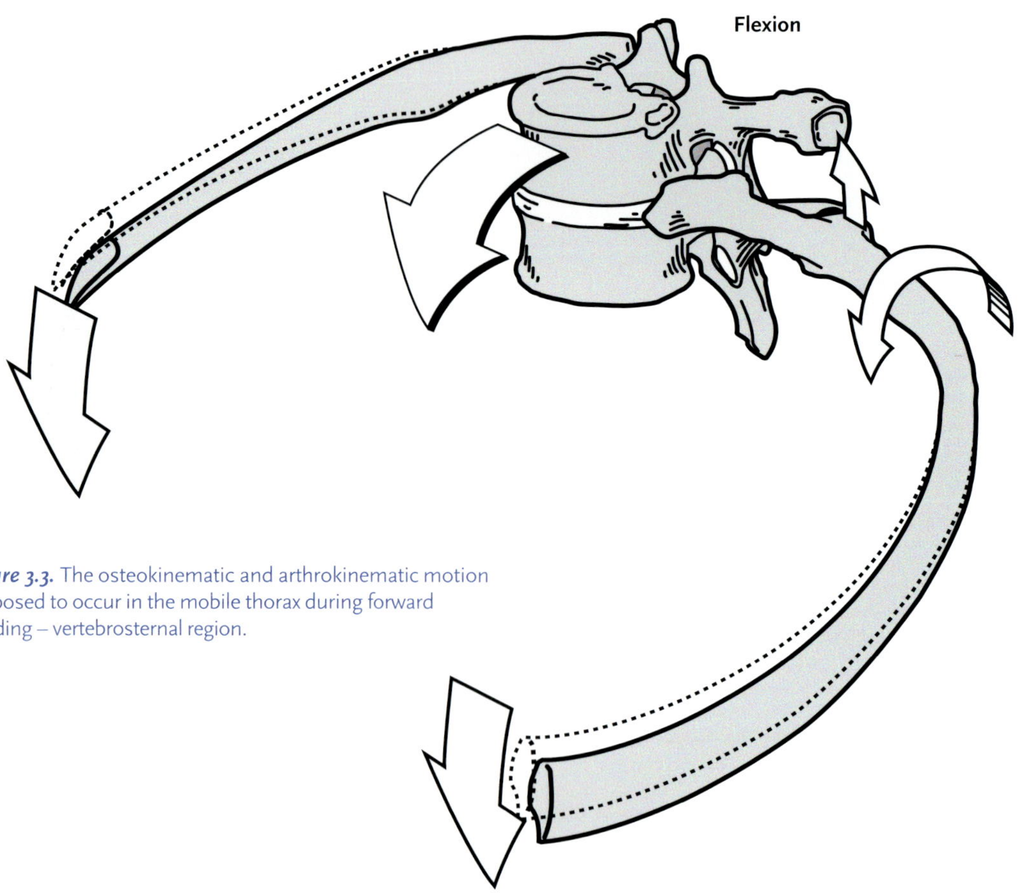

Figure 3.3. The osteokinematic and arthrokinematic motion proposed to occur in the mobile thorax during forward bending – vertebrosternal region.

considerable independent movement of the sternum and the spine is possible, "thus allowing mobility of the spine without forcing concomitant movements of (the) rib cage". This is supported clinically in that three movement patterns are apparent in this region of the thorax and depend on the relative flexibility between the spinal column and the rib cage. In the very young, (less than 12 years of age) the head of the rib does not fully articulate with the inferior aspect of the superior vertebra (Williams et al 1989). In other words, the superior costovertebral joint is not completely developed prior to puberty. The secondary ossification centres for the head of the rib do not develop until puberty; therefore, the young chest is much more mobile. In the skeletally mature, the superior costovertebral joints limit the degree of rotation possible in all three planes. In old age, the costal cartilages tend to ossify superficially and decrease the pliability and relative flexibility of the thorax. This change in relative flexibility is apparent when examining the specific costal osteokinematics during forward/backward bending of trunk.

1. During flexion of the mobile thorax (Fig. 3.3), flexion of the superior vertebra occurs. The ribs anteriorly rotate about a paracoronal axis along the line of the neck of the rib such that the anterior aspect travels inferiorly while the posterior aspect travels superiorly. At the limit

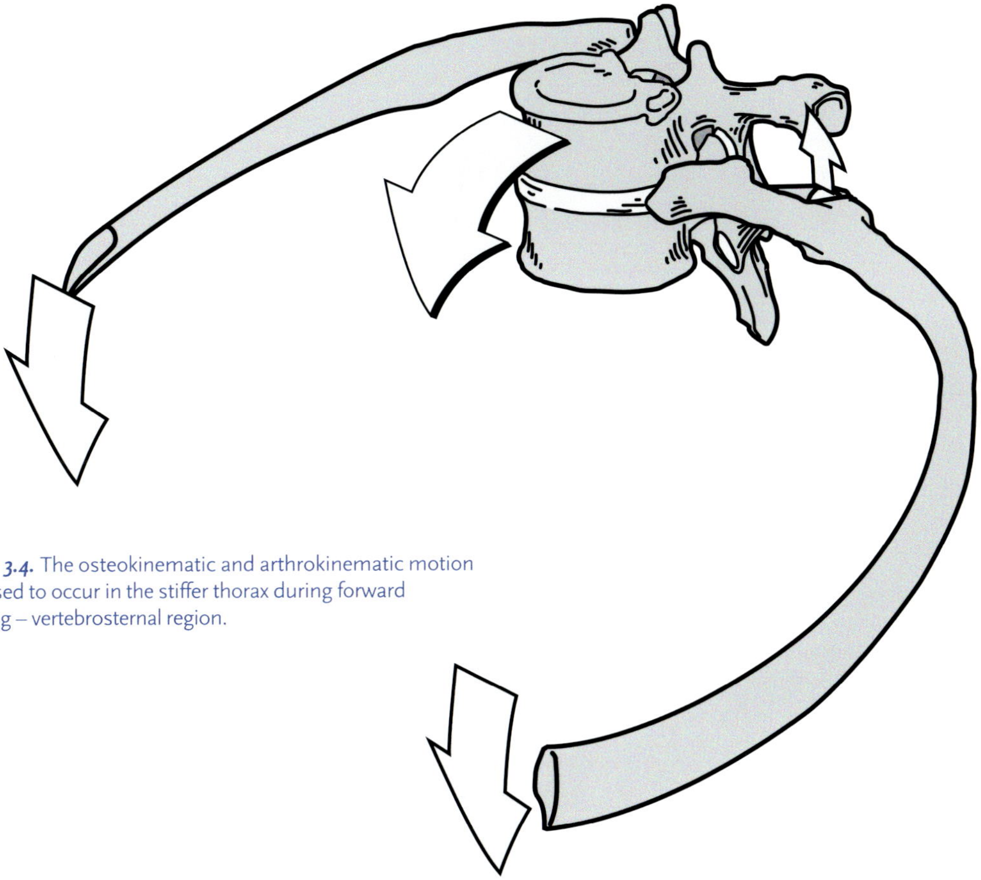

Figure 3.4. The osteokinematic and arthrokinematic motion proposed to occur in the stiffer thorax during forward bending – vertebrosternal region.

of forward bending, the vertebrae stop and the ribs continue to anteriorly rotate relative to the vertebrae.

Arthrokinematically, the inferior facets of the superior thoracic vertebra glide superoanteriorly at the zygapophyseal joints. The superior articular processes of the inferior thoracic vertebra present a gentle curve convex posterior in both the sagittal and coronal plane. The superior motion of the inferior articular processes follows the curve of this convexity and the result is a superoanterior glide. The anterior rotation of the rib results in a superior glide coupled with an anterior roll of the tubercle at the costotransverse joint.

2. In the stiff thorax (Fig. 3.4), the ribs are less flexible than the spinal column. During flexion, the anterior aspect of the rib travels inferiorly while the posterior aspect travels superiorly. Once the range of motion of the rib cage is exhausted, the thoracic vertebrae continue to flex on the now stationary ribs. The arthrokinematics of the zygapophyseal joints remain a superoanterior glide. At the costotransverse joints, the arthrokinematics are different. As the thoracic vertebrae continue to forward flex, the concave facets on the transverse processes travel superiorly relative to the tubercle of the ribs. The result is a relative inferior glide coupled with a posterior roll of the tubercle of the rib at the costotransverse joint.

3. The third movement pattern occurs when the relative flexibility between the spinal column and the rib cage is the same. During flexion of the thorax, the quantity of movement is reduced and there is no apparent movement between the thoracic vertebrae and the ribs. Some superoanterior gliding occurs at the zygapophyseal joints, however very little, if any, costotransverse joint motion can be felt.

Extension

Extension of the thoracic vertebra occurs during backward bending of the trunk and during bilateral elevation of the arms. Panjabi et al (1976) found that extension around the X axis coupled with posterior translation along the Z axis and very slight distraction (Fig. 3.5). When backward translation along the Z axis was induced in the experimental model, extension around the X axis and very slight compression also occurred.

The osteokinematic motion of the ribs which occurs during extension of the thoracic vertebra was not noted in either study by Panjabi et al (1976) or Willems et al (1996). Clinically, the movement patterns observed appear once again to depend on relative flexibility between the spinal column and the rib cage. Three patterns have been noted.

1. During extension of the mobile thorax (Fig. 3.6), extension of the superior vertebra occurs. The ribs posteriorly rotate about a paracoronal axis along the line of the neck of the rib such that the anterior aspect travels superiorly while the posterior aspect travels inferiorly. At the limit of backward bending, the vertebrae stop and the ribs continue to posteriorly rotate relative to the vertebrae.

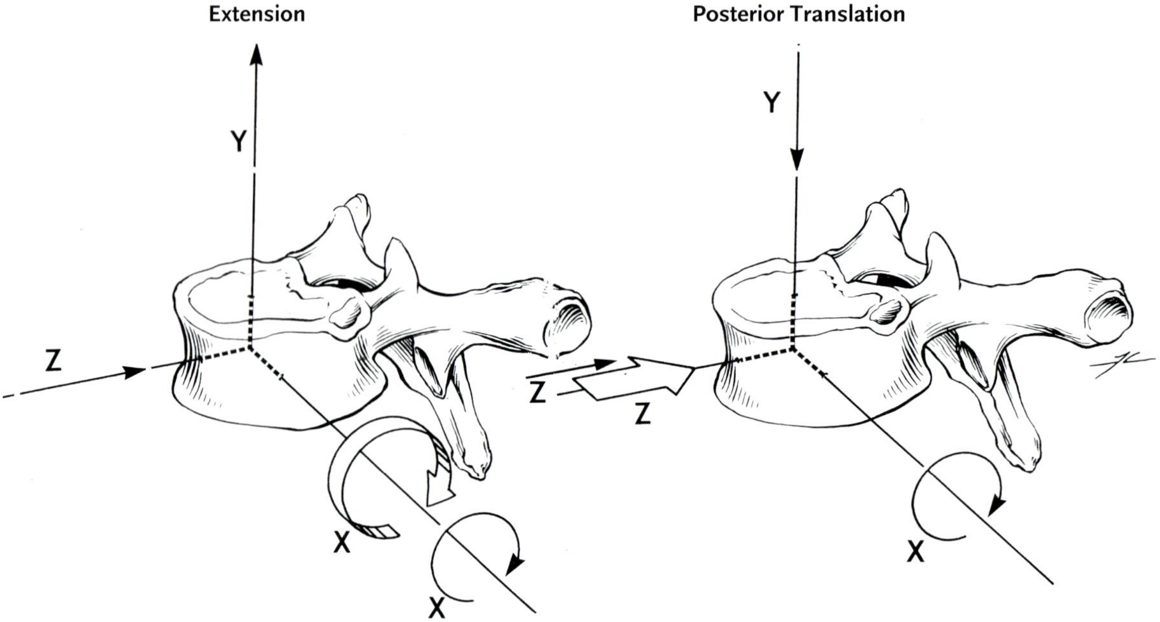

Figure 3.5. Extension around the X axis induced posterior translation along the Z axis and slight distraction along the Y axis. Posterior translation along the Z axis induced backward sagittal rotation around the X axis and slight compression along the Y axis (Panjabi et al 1976).

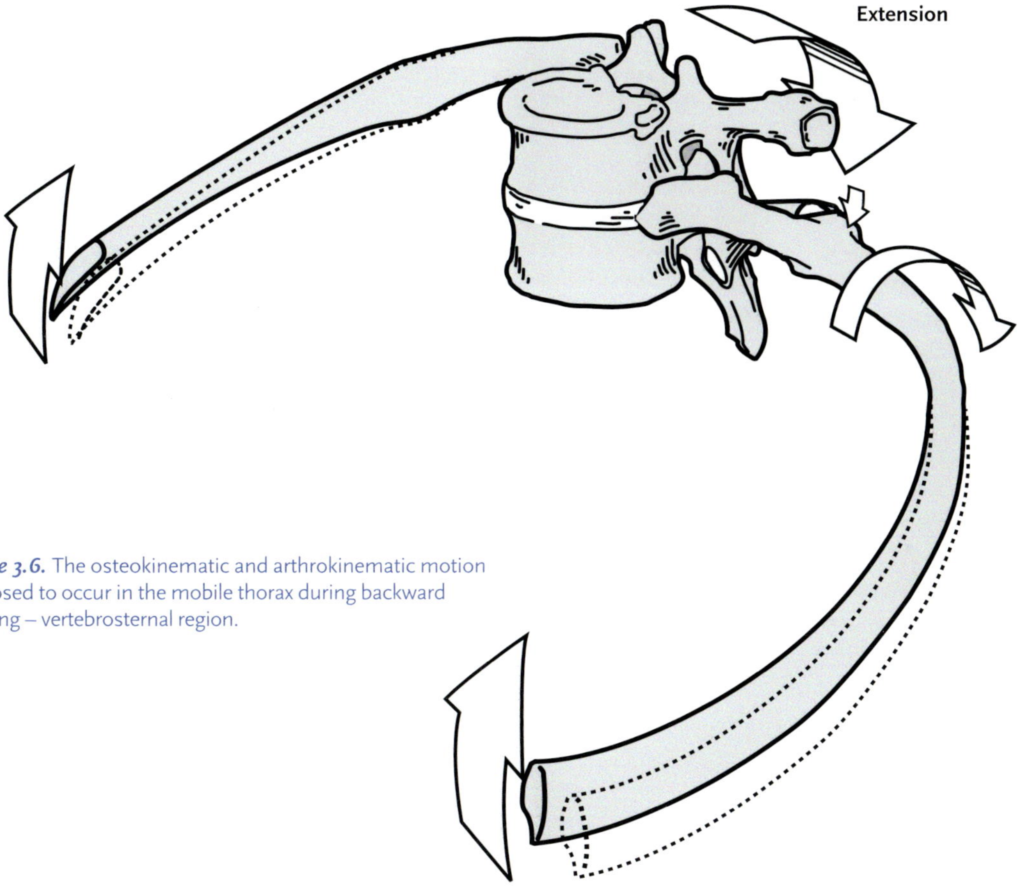

Figure 3.6. The osteokinematic and arthrokinematic motion proposed to occur in the mobile thorax during backward bending – vertebrosternal region.

Arthrokinematically, the inferior facets of the superior thoracic vertebra glide inferoposteriorly at the zygapophyseal joints. The superior articular processes present a gentle curve convex posterior in both the sagittal and coronal plane. The inferior motion of the inferior articular processes follows the curve of this convexity and the result is an inferoposterior glide. The posterior rotation of the neck of the rib results in an inferior glide coupled with a posterior roll of the tubercle at the costotransverse joint.

2. During extension of the stiff thorax (Fig. 3.7), the ribs are less flexible than the spinal column. Initially, the anterior aspect of the rib travels superiorly while the posterior aspect travels inferiorly. Once the range of motion of the rib cage is exhausted, the thoracic vertebrae continue to extend on the now stationary ribs. The arthrokinematics of the zygapophyseal joints remain an inferoposterior glide. At the costotransverse joints, the arthrokinematics are different. As the thoracic vertebrae continue to extend, the concave facets on the transverse processes travel inferiorly relative to the tubercle of the ribs. The result is a relative superior glide coupled with an anterior roll of the tubercle of the rib at the costotransverse joint.

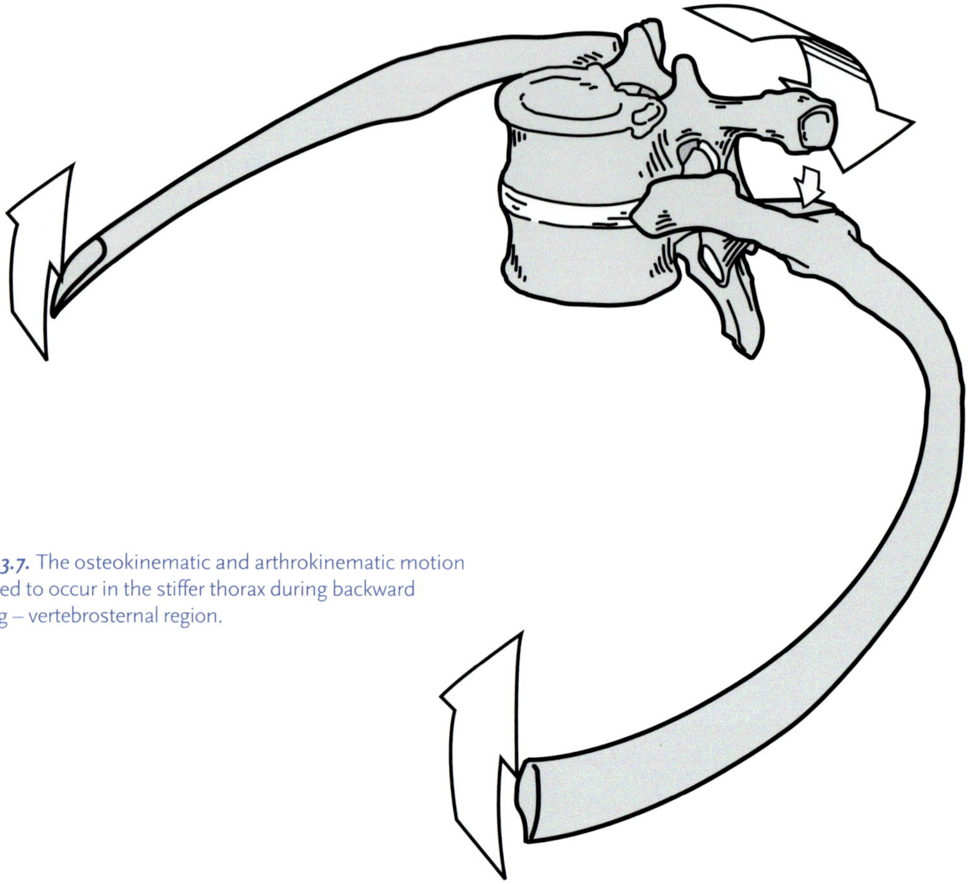

Figure 3.7. The osteokinematic and arthrokinematic motion proposed to occur in the stiffer thorax during backward bending – vertebrosternal region.

3. The third movement pattern occurs when the relative flexibility between the spinal column and the rib cage is the same. During extension of the thorax, the quantity of movement is reduced and there is no apparent movement between the thoracic vertebrae and the ribs. Some inferoposterior gliding occurs at the zygapophyseal joints only, however very little, if any, costotransverse joint motion can be felt.

These are the common patterns noted when sagittal plane motion of the thorax is observed. It is possible for individuals to voluntarily change their pattern of motion. For example, in the mobile thorax the spine can extend inducing a posterior rotation of the ribs in space and then while holding this position, it is possible to anteriorly rotate the ribs. This flexibility allows the thorax to accommodate the demands coming from

- respiration,
- movements of the upper extremities and
- movements of the head.

Lateral bending

Sideflexion of the thoracic vertebrae occurs during lateral bending of the trunk. Panjabi et al (1976) found that sideflexion, or rotation around the Z axis, coupled with contralateral rotation around the Y axis and ipsilateral translation along the X axis (Fig. 3.8). Translation along the X axis coupled with ipsilateral sideflexion around the Z axis and contralateral rotation around the Y axis.

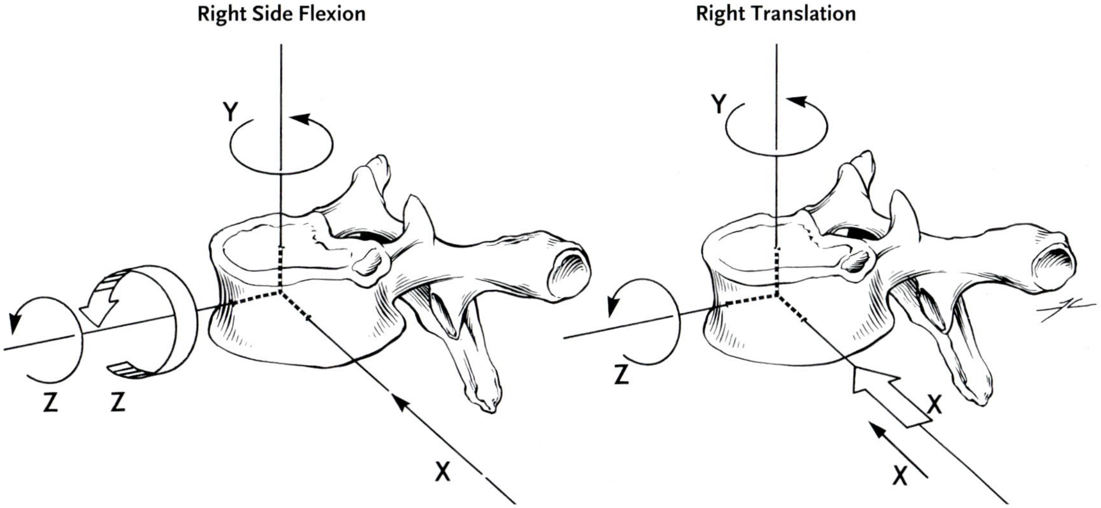

Figure 3.8. Right sideflexion around the Z axis induced left rotation around the Y axis and right translation along the X axis. Right lateral translation along the X axis induced right sideflexion around the Z axis and left rotation around the Y axis (Panjabi et al 1976).

Willems et al's (1996) found that the pattern of coupling during lateral bending was variable, although an ipsilateral relationship predominated. Since the movement of the sensor was only compared to its baseline starting position, the pattern noted in this study can only reflect how the spinous process moved in space and no comment can be made on segmental motion patterning. In other words, during lateral bending of the trunk, Willems et al (1996) noted that the vertebra tended to sideflex and rotate in an ipsilateral direction. Sideflex and rotate compared to what? No comment can be made on what T4 did relative to T5 because this was not measured. In this study, T4 sideflexed and rotated in an ipsilateral direction (compared to its starting position) during lateral bending of the thorax. If T5 rotated more than T4, then the resultant segmental motion would, in fact, be a contralateral rotation.

It is interesting to postulate on what produces coupled motion in the thorax. In the midcervical spine, it is thought (Penning & Wilmink 1987) that the oblique orientation of the zygapophyseal joints together with the uncinate processes directs the ipsilateral rotation and sideflexion which occurs. In the lumbar spine, the zygapophyseal

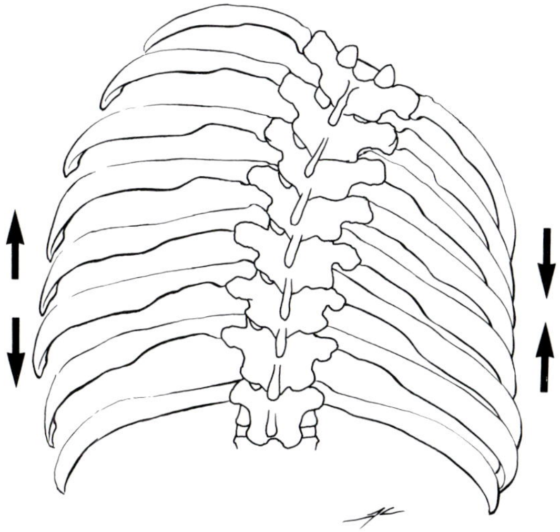

Figure 3.9. As the thorax sideflexes to the right, the ribs on the right approximate and the ribs on the left separate at their lateral margins. The costal motion stops first, the thoracic vertebrae then continue to sideflex slightly to the right.

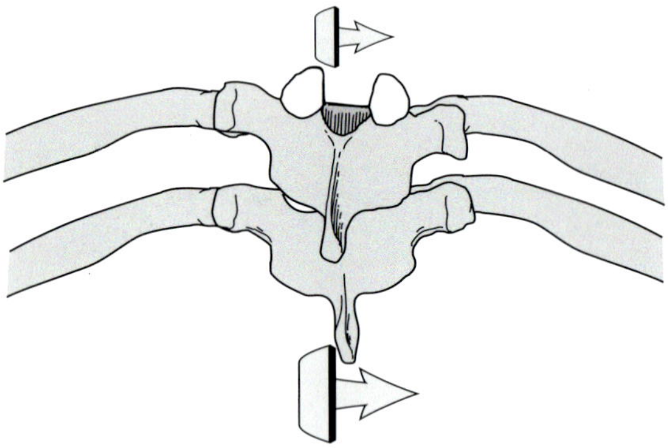

Figure 3.10. Since the tubercle of the rib is convex, as the thoracic vertebra sideflexes to the right it has to move posterior and inferior on the right and anterior and superior on the left. Osteokinematically, this produces a right rotation of the thoracic vertebra relative to its starting position. As T5 sideflexes to the right on the fixed 5th ribs, it rotates to the right (necessitated by the shape of the tubercle of the 5th ribs). T4 follows this motion, however the relative anterior rotation of the right 5th rib and posterior rotation of the left 5th rib limit the amplitude of the right rotation of T4 such that it rotates less to the right than T5 and is therefore relatively left rotated. This only occurs at the limit of lateral bending.

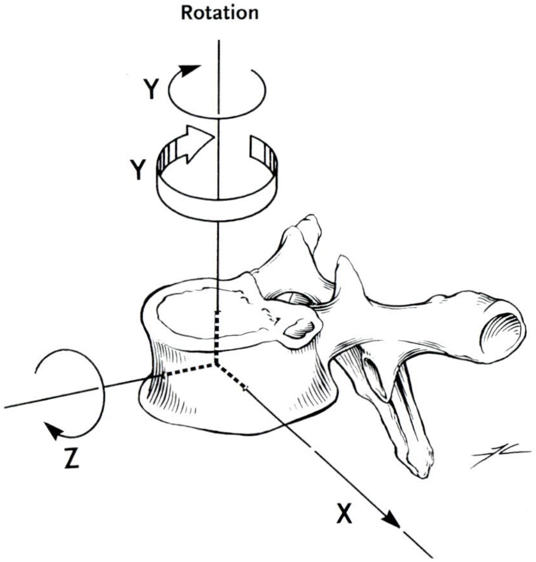

Figure 3.11. Panjabi et al (1976) found that right rotation around the Y axis induced left sideflexion around the Z axis and left translation along the X axis.

joints also are known (Bogduk 1997) to influence the direction of motion coupling during rotation. However, the facets of the zygapophyseal joints in the thoracic spine lie in a somewhat coronal plane and would not limit pure sideflexion during lateral bending of the trunk. It is difficult to see how they could be responsible for the rotation (ipsilateral or contralateral) found to occur during sideflexion.

As the trunk bends laterally to the right, a left convex curve is produced. The thoracic vertebrae sideflex to the right and the ribs on the right approximate while the ribs on the left separate at their lateral margins (Fig. 3.9). In both the mobile thorax and the stiff thorax, the ribs appear to stop moving before the thoracic vertebrae. The thoracic vertebrae then continue to sideflex to the right. This motion can be palpated at the costotransverse joint.

This slight increase in right sideflexion of the thoracic vertebrae against the fixed ribs is proposed to cause the following arthrokinematic motion. At the costotransverse joints, a relative superior glide of the tubercle of the right rib and a relative inferior glide of the tubercle of the left rib occurs as the vertebra continues to sideflex to the right against the fixed ribs (Fig. 3.10). Since the costotransverse joint is concavoconvex in a sagittal plane, the superior glide of the right rib produces a relative anterior roll of the neck of the rib with respect to the transverse process (remember that the rib is stationary and the moving bone is actually the thoracic vertebra). The inferior glide of the left rib produces a posterior roll of the neck of the rib relative to the transverse process. Again, it is important to note that the moving bone is the thoracic vertebra, not the rib. Since the tubercle of the rib is convex, as the thoracic vertebra sideflexes to the right it has to move posterior and inferior on the right and anterior and superior on the left. Osteokinematically, this produces a right rotation of the thoracic vertebra relative to its starting position. This is exactly what Willems et al (1996) found in their study. However, consider what happens not just in space, but between two thoracic vertebrae. As T5 sideflexes to the right on the fixed 5th ribs, it rotates to the right (necessitated by the shape of the tubercle of the 5th ribs). T4 follows this motion; however the head of the rib limits the amplitude of the right rotation of T4 such that it rotates less to the right than T5 and is therefore relatively left rotated. This only occurs at the limit of lateral bending.

In summary, during lateral bending of the vertebrosternal region, the vertebrae sideflex and rotate ipsilaterally relative to their starting position. Relative to one another, the superior vertebra rotates less than the level below and therefore is actually left rotated in comparison. This coupling of motion only occurs at the end of the range. In the mid-position, either ipsilateral or contralateral coupling can occur.

Panjabi et al (1976) found that right lateral translation along the X axis occurred during right sideflexion (Fig. 3.8). The effect of this right lateral translation is negated by the left lateral translation which occurs as the superior vertebra rotates to the left. The net effect is minimal, if any, lateral translation of the ribs along the line of the neck of the rib at the costotransverse joints. The clinical impression is that no anteromedial or posterolateral slide of the ribs occurs during lateral bending of the trunk.

At the zygapophyseal joints, the left inferior articular process of the superior thoracic vertebra glides superoanteromedially and the right glides inferoposterolaterally to facilitate right sideflexion and left rotation of the superior vertebra.

Rotation

Panjabi et al (1976) found that rotation around the Y axis coupled with contralateral rotation around the Z axis and contralateral translation along the X axis (Fig. 3.11). This is not consistent with clinical observation (Fig. 3.12). In the midthoracic spine, rotation around the Y axis has been found to be coupled with ipsilateral rotation around the Z axis and contralateral translation along the X axis. In other words, when axial rotation is the first motion induced, rotation and sideflexion appear to occur to the same side in the midthoracic spine. Willems et al's (1996) found intersubject variation in motion patterning when the primary movement was axial rotation, however an ipsilateral relationship was predominant. It may be that the thorax must be intact and stable both anteriorly and posteriorly for this in vivo coupling of motion to occur. The anterior elements of the thorax were removed 3 cm lateral to the costotransverse joints in the study by Panjabi et

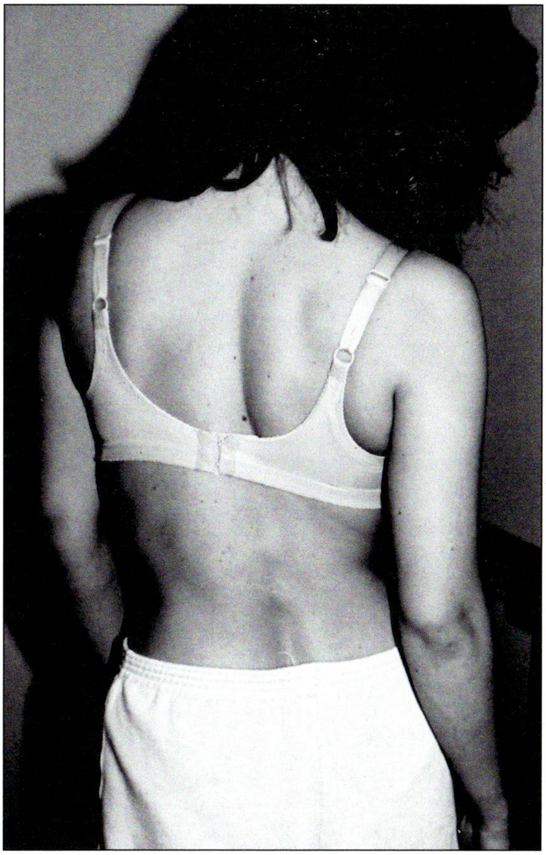

Figure 3.12. Clinically, the midthorax appears to sideflex and rotate to the same side during rotation of the trunk.

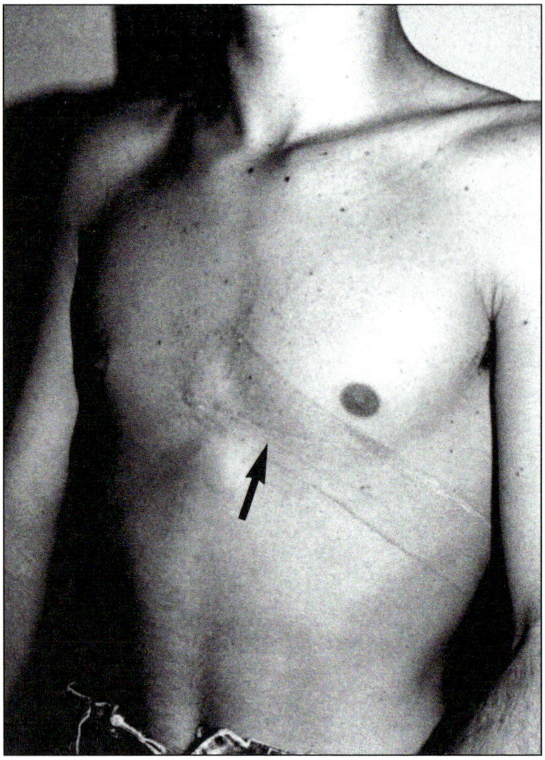

Figure 3.13a The costocartilage of the left sixth rib was removed (arrow points to the incision) in this seventeen year old.

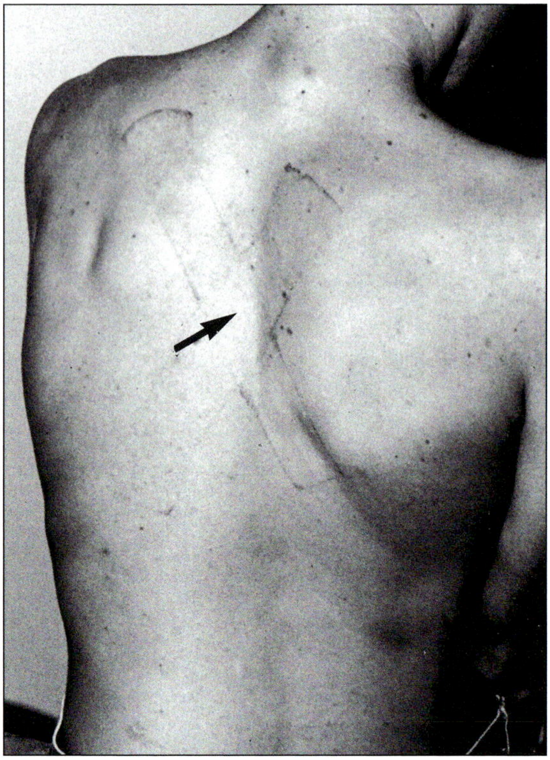

Figure 3.13b. Note the inability of the midthorax to rotate and sideflex to the right during right rotation of the trunk (arrow). Instability prevents the normal biomechanics of ipsilateral sideflexion/ rotation during rotation of the trunk.

al. When the anterior elements of the thorax are removed surgically, ipsilateral sideflexion and rotation cannot occur in the midthorax. The seventeen year old youth illustrated in Figures 3.13a,b had the costocartilage of the left sixth rib removed for cosmetic reasons. Subsequently, he presented with persistent pain in the midthorax and on examination of axial rotation contralateral sideflexion occurred at the 6th segment.

During right rotation of the trunk the following biomechanics are proposed to occur in the midthorax. The superior vertebra (eg. T5) rotates to the right and translates to the left (Fig. 3.14). The left (6th) rib anteriorly rotates and translates posterolateral relative to the ipsilateral transverse process of the inferior vertebra (T6) and the right (6th) rib posteriorly rotates and translates anteromedial relative to the ipsilateral transverse process of the inferior vertebra (T6).

When the limit of this horizontal translation is reached, both the costovertebral and the costotransverse ligaments are tensed. Stability of the ribs both anteriorly and posteriorly is required for the following motion to occur. Further right rotation of the superior vertebra (T5) occurs as the superior vertebral body tilts to the right (glides superiorly along the left superior costovertebral joint and inferiorly along the right superior costovertebral joint). This tilt causes right sideflexion of the superior vertebra (T5-6) during right rotation of the midthoracic segment (Fig. 3.15).

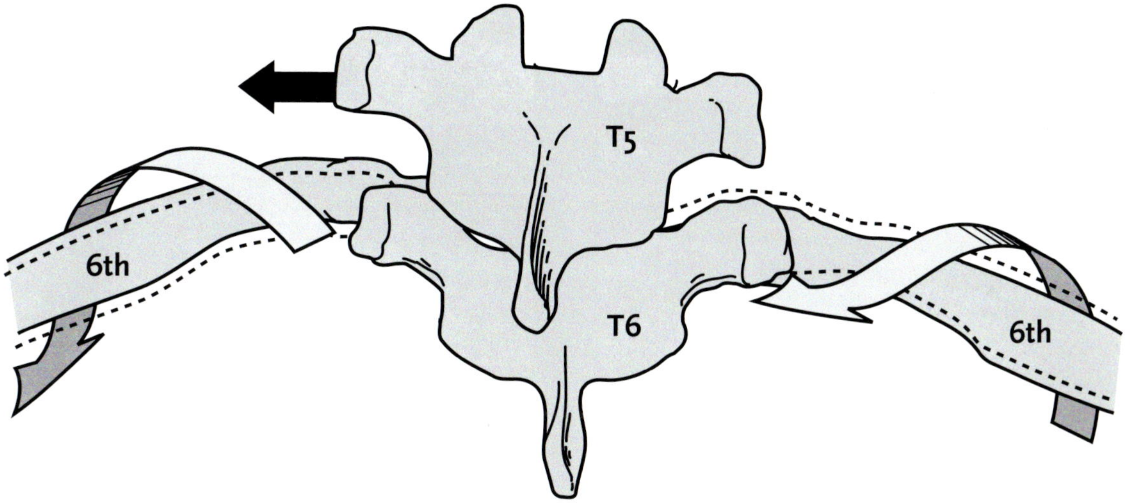

Figure 3.14. The osteokinematic and arthrokinematic motion proposed to occur in the vertebrosternal region during right rotation of the trunk.

At the zygapophyseal joints, the left inferior articular process of the superior vertebra glides superolaterally, the right inferior articular process glides inferomedially to facilitate right rotation and right sideflexion of the thoracic vertebra.

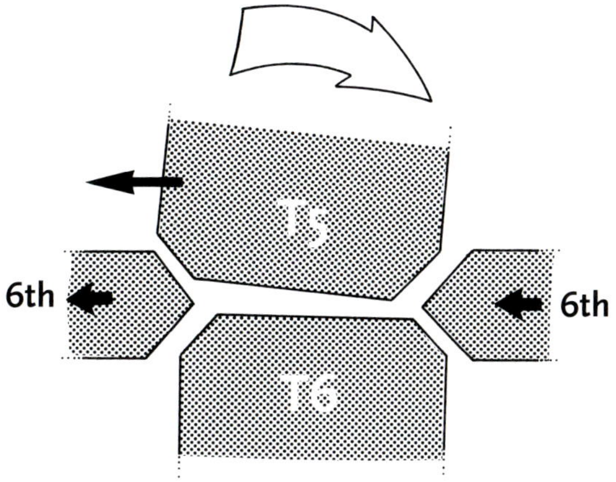

Figure 3.15. At the limit of left lateral translation, the superior vertebra sideflexes to the right along the plane of the pseudo 'U' joint (analogous to the uncovertebral joint of the midcervical spine) formed by the intervertebral disc and the superior costovertebral joints.

Vertebrochondral Region

There are significant differences in the anatomy of this region that subsequently influence the biomechanics. The facets on the transverse processes of the lower thoracic vertebrae are more planar and oriented in a superolateral direction (Williams et al 1989). A superoinferior glide of the rib will therefore not necessarily be associated with the same degree of anteroposterior rotation found in the vertebrosternal region. The costocartilages of the ribs seven to ten are less firmly attached to the sternum. The inferior demifacet on the body of T9 for the 10th rib is small and often absent. The 10th rib articulates with one facet on the body of T10 and often does not attach to the transverse process at all.

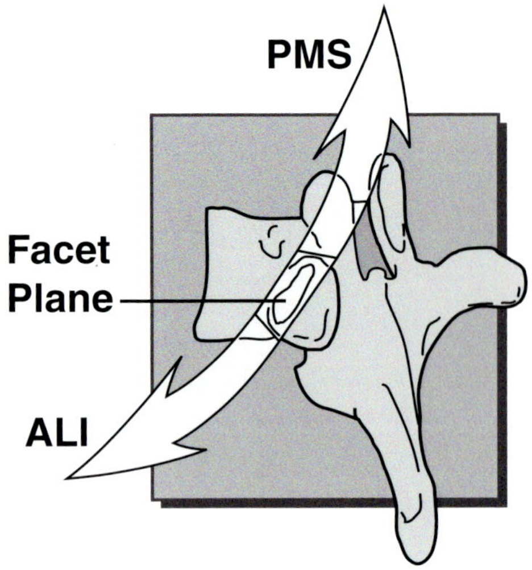

Figure 3.16. The plane of the costotransverse joint in the vertebrochondral region – posteromediosuperior (a glide in this direction occurs during anterior rotation of the rib) and anterolateroinferior (a glide in this direction occurs during posterior rotation of the rib).

Flexion/extension

Flexion of the thoracic vertebrae in this region occurs during forward bending of the trunk. Clinically, it appears that the associated ribs follow the sagittal motion although minimal articular motion is necessary at the costovertebral joints of ribs 9 and 10 since they do not have a large attachment to the superior vertebra. The zygapophyseal joints glide superiorly during flexion and inferiorly in extension.

Lateral bending

The biomechanics of the vertebrochondral region during lateral bending of the trunk depend on the apex of the curve produced in sideflexion. For example, if during right lateral bending of the trunk the apex of the sideflexion curve is at the level of the greater trochanter on the left, then all of the thoracic vertebrae will sideflex to the right, the ribs will approximate on the right and separate on the left. As the rib cage is compressed on the right and stops moving, further right sideflexion of the vertebrochondral region will result in a superior glide of the ribs at the costotransverse joints on the right. Given the orientation of the articular surfaces (Fig. 3.16), the glide that occurs is posteromediosuperior on the right and anterolateroinferior on the left with minimal, if any, rotation of the neck of the rib. The ribs do not appear to direct the superior vertebra into contralateral rotation as they do in the verte-

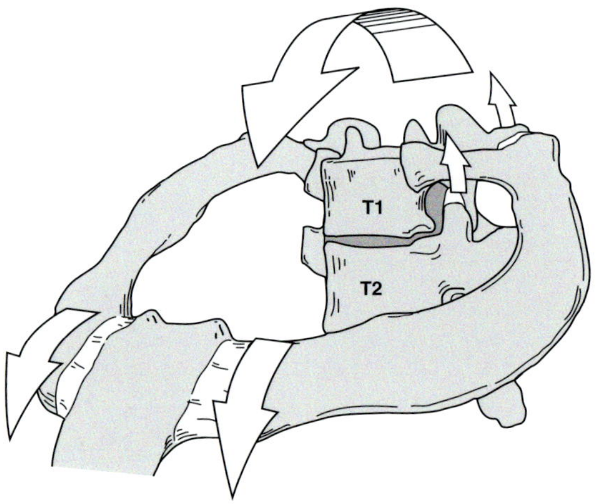

Figure 3.17. The osteokinematic and arthrokinematic motion proposed to occur in the vertebromanubrial region during forward bending.

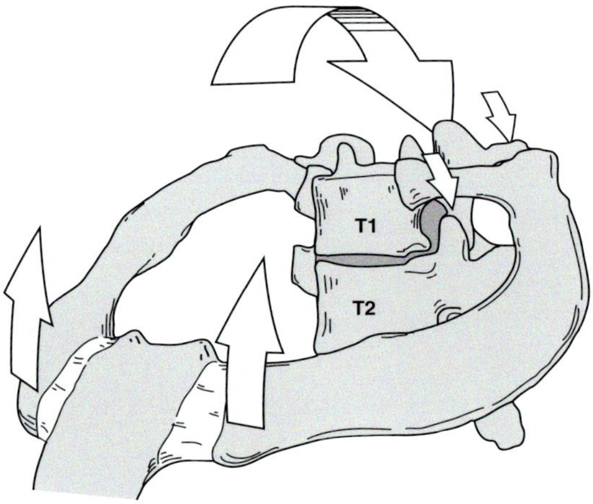

Figure 3.18. The osteokinematic and arthrokinematic motion proposed to occur in the vertebromanubrial region during bilateral elevation of the arms.

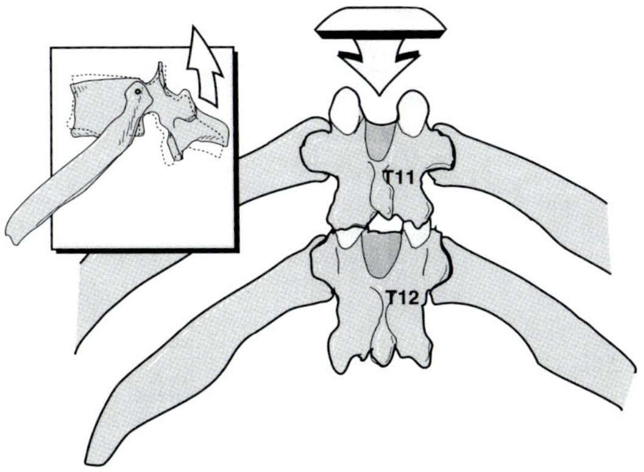

Figure 3.19. The osteokinematic and arthrokinematic motion proposed to occur in the thoracolumbar region during forward bending.

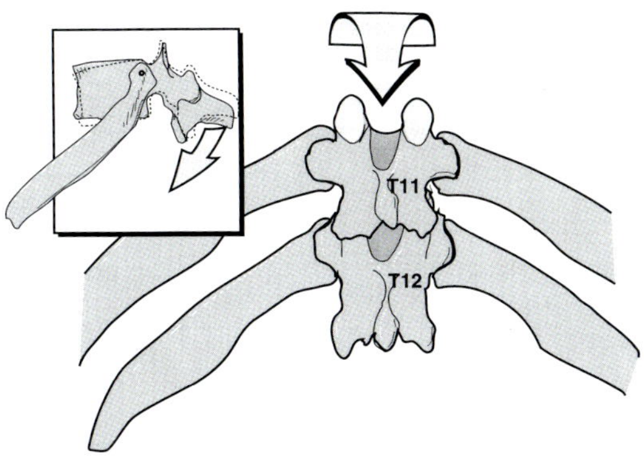

Figure 3.20. The osteokinematic and arthrokinematic motion proposed to occur in the thoracolumbar region during backward bending.

brosternal region. The vertebrae are then free to follow the rotation that is congruent with the levels above and below.

If however, the apex of the sideflexion curve is within the thorax, (i.e. at T8), then the osteokinematics of the lower thoracic vertebrae appear to be very different. The rib cage remains compressed on the right and separated on the left, however, the thoracic vertebrae sideflex to the left below the apex of the right sideflexion curve (i.e. T9, T10, T11, T12). Given the orientation of the articular surfaces of the costotransverse joints, the glide that occurs on the right is in an anterolateroinferior direction (posteromediosuperior on the left) with minimal, if any, rotation of the neck of the rib. Once again, the ribs do not appear to direct the superior vertebra to rotate in a sense incongruent to the levels above and below.

Rotation

The same flexibility of motion coupling is apparent in the vertebrochondral region when rotation is considered. In fact, this region appears to be designed to rotate with minimal restriction from the costal elements. The coupled movement pattern for rotation here can be ipsilateral sideflexion or contralateral sideflexion. The coronally oriented facets of the zygapophyseal joints do not dictate a coupling of sideflexion when rotation is induced. The small superior costovertebral joint and the lack of a direct anterior attachment of the associated ribs facilitates this flexibility in motion patterning.

Vertebromanubrial and Thoracolumbar Region

Flexion/Extension

The first two ribs are always less mobile than T1 or T2 and the movement pattern for flexion (Fig. 3.17) and extension (Fig. 3.18) in the vertebromanubrial region is consistent with the stiff thorax pattern described in the vertebrosternal section. In the thoracolumbar region (Figs. 3.19, 3.20), the eleventh and twelfth costovertebral joints are unmodified ovoid in shape and flexion/extension of the thoracic vertebra can be a pure spin (MacConaill & Basmajian 1977).

Lateral bending

In the vertebromanubrial region, the head of the first rib does not articulate with C7 and the superoinferior glide of the ribs and the conjunct rotation which occurs cannot influence the direction of movement coupling between C7 and T1. C7-T1 and T1-T2 follow the same pattern of motion coupling as the midcervical spine when the head is bent laterally (Fig. 3.21). Sideflexion is coupled with ipsilateral rotation of the superior vertebra. The uncinate processes at C7-T1 may influence the direction of motion coupling here. During right lateral bending of the head/neck the transverse process glides inferiorly relative to the rib on the right and superiorly relative to the rib on the left.

At the thoracolumbar junction, pure sideflexion can occur. The heads of the eleventh and twelfth ribs do not articulate with the vertebra above and there is no costotransverse joint to consider. The costovertebral joint shape is an unmodified ovoid and therefore pure sideflexion of the thoracic vertebrae between two fixed ribs can occur.

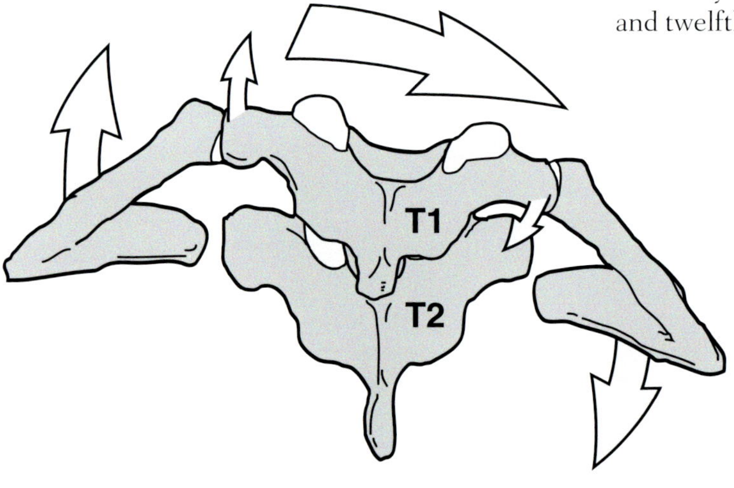

Figure 3.21. The osteokinematic and arthrokinematic motion proposed to occur in the vertebromanubrial region during lateral bending of the head to the right.

Rotation

In the vertebromanubrial region, C7-T1 and T1-T2 follow the same pattern of motion coupling as the midcervical spine when the head is rotated. Rotation is coupled with ipsilateral sideflexion of the superior vertebra. The two uncinate processes at C7-T1 may influence the direction of motion coupling here. During right rotation of the head/neck the transverse process glides inferiorly relative to the rib on the right and superiorly relative to the rib on the left.

Considerable flexibility of motion coupling is apparent in the thoracolumbar junction. Anatomically, the lower thoracic levels (T10, T11) are designed to rotate with minimal restriction from the ribs. Passively, the T11-12 segment can be purely rotated about a vertical axis with no restriction from the zygapophyseal joints or the ribs. Actively, the coupled movement pattern for rotation in this region can be ipsilateral sideflexion or contralateral sideflexion. The coronally oriented facets of the zygapophyseal joints do not dictate a specific coupling of sideflexion when rotation is induced. The absence of a costotransverse joint and the lack of a direct anterior attachment of the associated ribs facilitates this flexibility in motion patterning at the eleventh and twelfth segments.

RESPIRATION

The diaphragm is the most efficient respiratory muscle. Optimally, during inspiration, the diaphragm descends and pulls the central tendon inferiorly through the fixed twelfth ribs and L1 to L3. Osteokinematically, the lower ribs posteriorly rotate (arthrokinematic anterolateroinferior glide at the costotransverse joints) creating a lateral, anterior and posterior expansion of the rib cage. Further inspiration causes the vertebrosternal ribs to posteriorly rotate (arthrokinematic inferior glide with a posterior roll) further increasing the anteroposterior dimension of the thorax.

When motion of the lower ribs is limited by over-activation of the global system (oblique abdominals and erector spinae), lateral expansion of the thorax is limited and abdominal bulging (belly breathing) may result. Alternately, the chest expansion may be limited to the upper thorax (apical breathing). These breathing patterns are less optimal.

Expiration should occur passively as the diaphragm relaxes. The ribs anteriorly rotate and this requires a posteromediosuperior glide at the costotransverse joints of the vertebrochondral region and a superior glide/anterior roll at the costotransverse joints of the vertebrosternal region.

SUMMARY

The known biomechanics of the intact thorax continues to be far from complete. Willems et al (1996) acknowledge that "altered tension in muscles may change forces on the ribs and vertebrae which could in turn influence the pattern of coupled motion in vivo, particularly in the upper thoracic area". Inclusion criteria for studies such as these should involve a biomechanical examination and not just exclusion by lack of symptoms or history of problems since "it is not uncommon to find tightness in muscles... even in asymptomatic persons" (Willems et al 1996). This is an excellent study and with further refinement of the inclusion criteria (biomechanical evaluation) and methodology (sensors on adjacent levels) could yield significant information pertinent to understanding the biomechanics of the thorax.

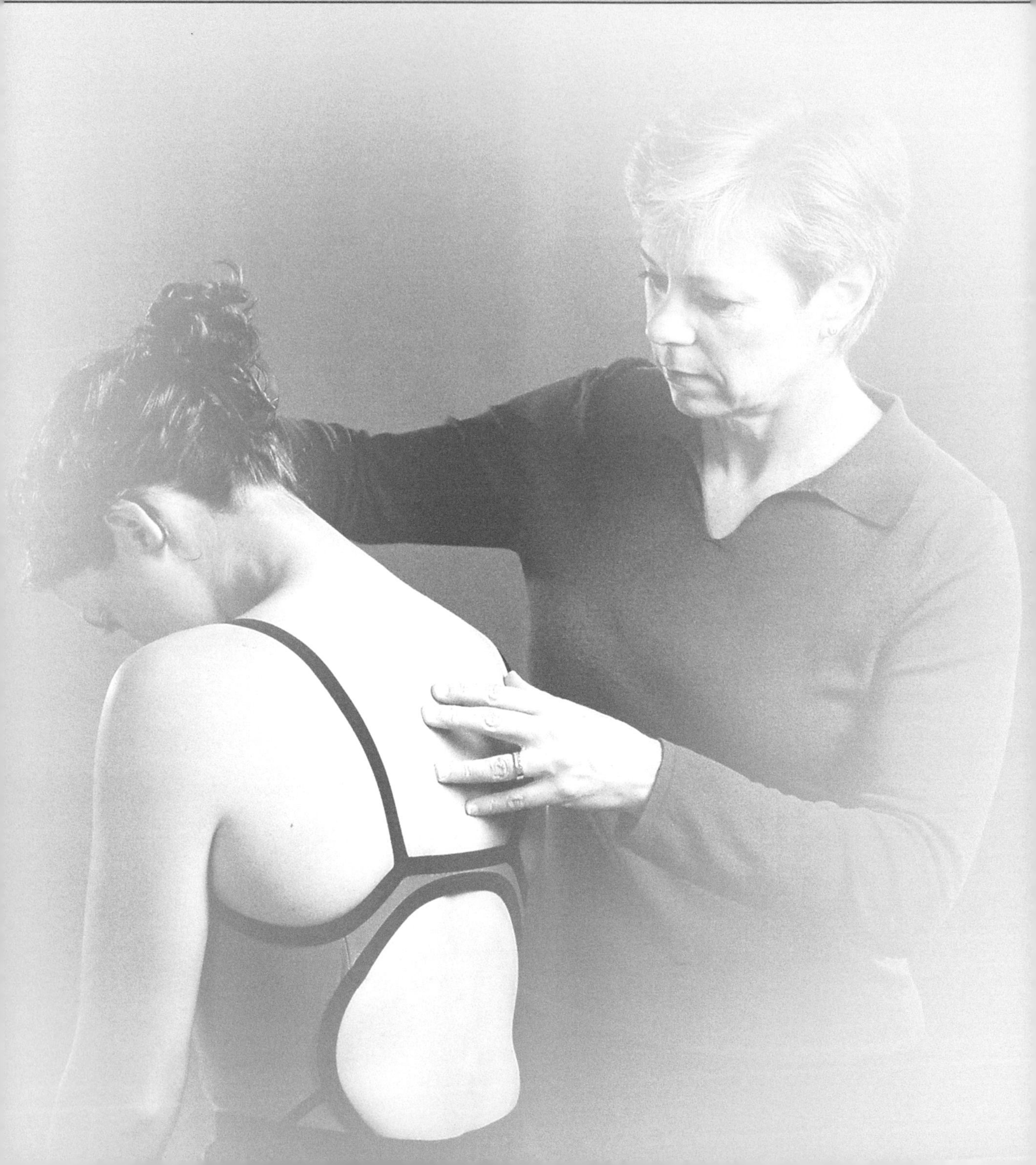

4

DIAGNOSING THE THORACIC DYSFUNCTION

Impaired thoracic function can be defined as an inability to effectively move and/or transfer forces through the thorax. To reach this diagnosis, specific functional tests for mobility and load transfer are required. To understand the underlying cause for the functional impairment, specific tests that examine form closure, force closure, motor control and the effect of negative emotional states are required.

The reader is referred to the CD-ROM which accompanies this text to view short video clips of these tests.

SUBJECTIVE EXAMINATION

The purpose of the subjective examination is to establish the nature, irritability and severity of the presenting problem (Table 1).

Mode of Onset

Was the onset of symptoms sudden or insidious? Was there an element of trauma? If so, was there a major traumatic event over a short period of time, such as a motor vehicle accident, or were there a series of minor traumatic events over a long period of time. Is the patient presenting during the acute, subacute or chronic (substrate, fibroblastic or maturation) phase of healing? Is this the first episode requiring treatment or is this a recurring problem?

Pain/Dysaesthesia

Where is the pain and/or dysaesthesia? Is it localized or diffuse? Where does it radiate to and can its quality be described? If there is symptom referral, does it tend to refer around the chest or through the chest? What activities, if any, aggravate the symptoms? How long does it take for this activity to produce symptoms? Which activities (including how much) provide relief?

Sleep

Are the symptoms interfering with sleep? What kind of bed is being slept in and what position is most frequently adopted? Does rest provide relief?

Occupation/Leisure activities/Sports

What level of physical activity does the patient consider their normal and essential for return to full function? What are the patient's goals from therapy?

General Information

How is the patient's general health? Is any medication being taken for this or any other condition? What are the results of any adjunctive diagnostic tests (i.e. X-rays, CT scan, MRI, laboratory tests)?

OBJECTIVE EXAMINATION

Impaired thoracic function can be defined as an inability to effectively move and/or transfer forces through the thorax. To reach this diagnosis, specific functional tests for mobility and load transfer are required. To understand the underlying cause for the functional impairment, specific tests that examine form closure, force closure, motor control and the effect of negative emotional states are required. The impact of the specific impairment is often reflected in the patient's posture and this is where the objective examination begins.

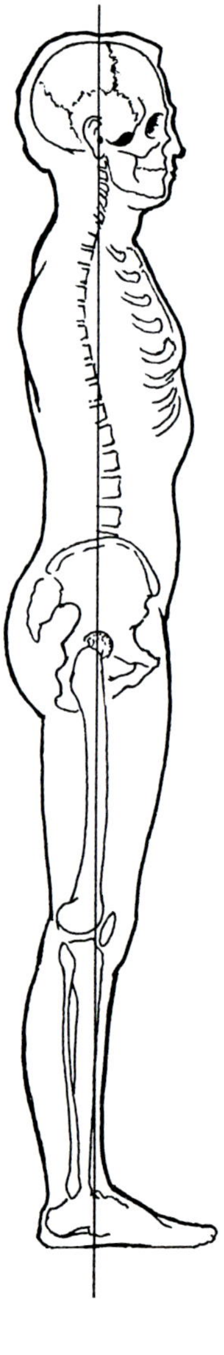

Figure 4.1 Optimal posture.

Postural Analysis

Optimal posture requires the following. In the sagittal plane, a vertical line should pass through the external auditory meatus, the bodies of the cervical vertebrae, the glenohumeral joint, slightly anterior to the bodies of the thoracic vertebrae transecting the vertebrae at the thoracolumbar junction, the bodies of the lumbar vertebrae, the sacral promontory, slightly posterior to the hip joint and slightly anterior to the talocrural joint and naviculo-calcaneo-cuboid joint (Fig. 4.1). The primary thoracic curve should be maintained i.e. no midthoracic lordosis.

In the coronal plane, the clavicles should be horizontal, the manubrium and sternum vertical (and in the same plane as the pubic symphysis and anterior superior iliac spines of the innominate) and the scapulae

Name	*Age*	*Dr.*
Current History: Mode of Onset		
Past History	*Past Treatment*	
Pain/Dysaesthesia		
Location	*Relieving Activities*	*Aggravating Activities*
Special Questions		
Distal paraesthesia	*Bowel/bladder symptoms*	*Effect of sustained Slump and/or neck flexion*
Sleep		
Surface/Position	*Status in a.m.*	*Night Wakening*
General Information		
Occupation/sport/hobbies	*Medication*	*Adjunctive Tests*

Table 1. Subjective Examination

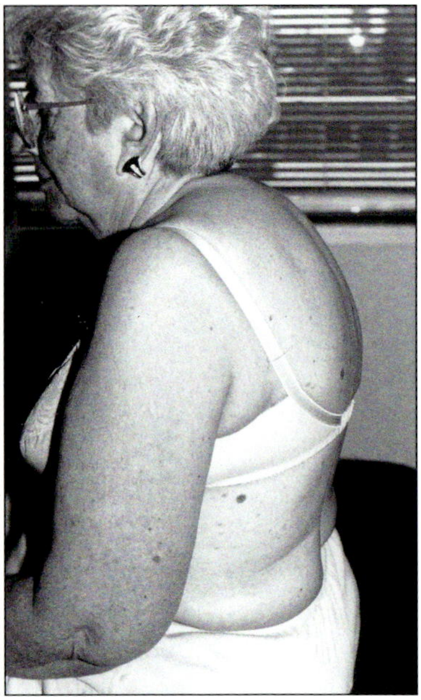

Figure 4.2 Excessive thoracic kyphosis secondary to osteoporosis.

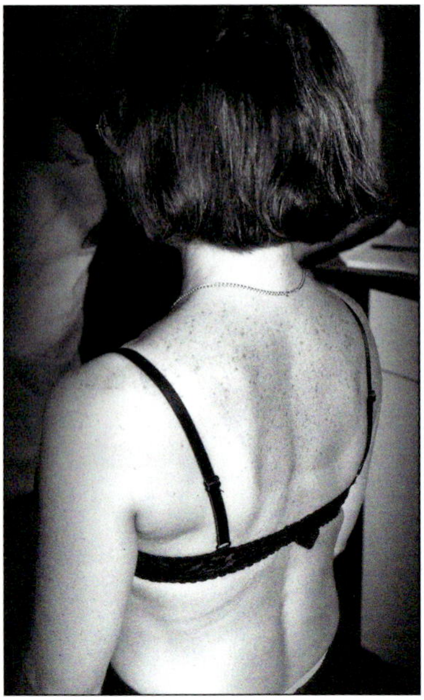

Figure 4.3 Excessive midthoracic lordosis secondary to overactivation of the global system of the thorax.

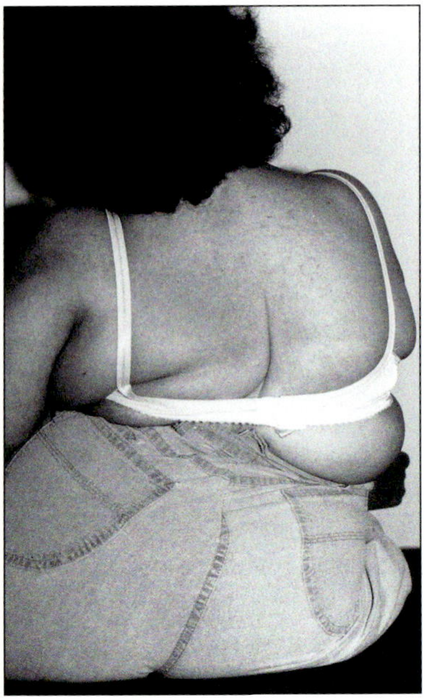

Figure 4.4 Excessive rotoscoliosis secondary to poliomyelitis and altered neural control of the local and global systems of the thorax.

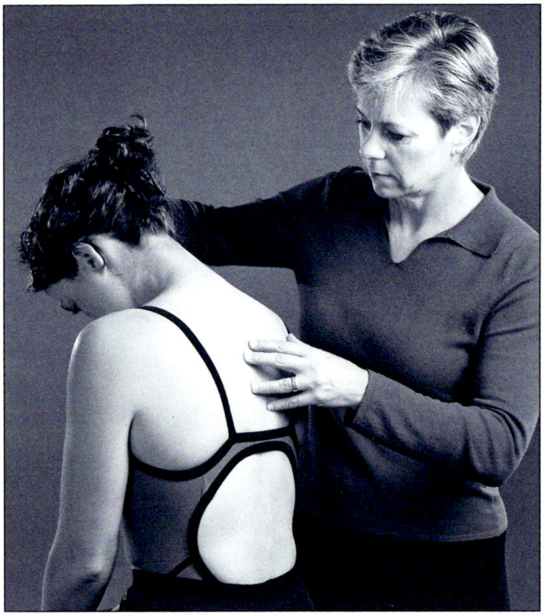

Figure 4.5 Functional movement testing – regional tests. Forward bending of the head.

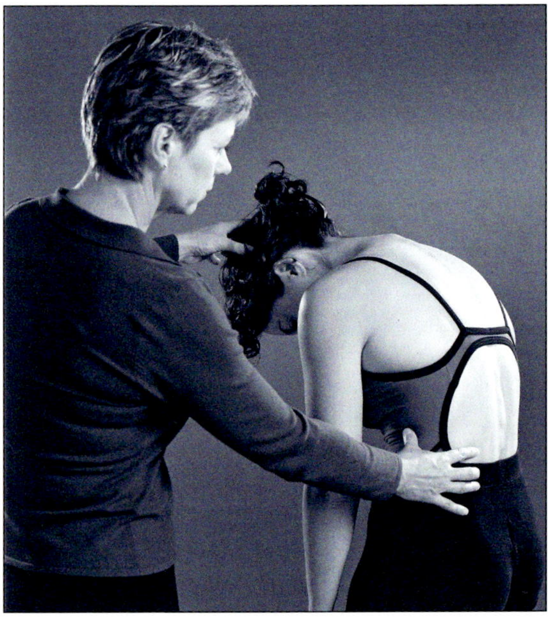

Figure 4.6 Functional movement testing – regional tests. Forward bending of the trunk.

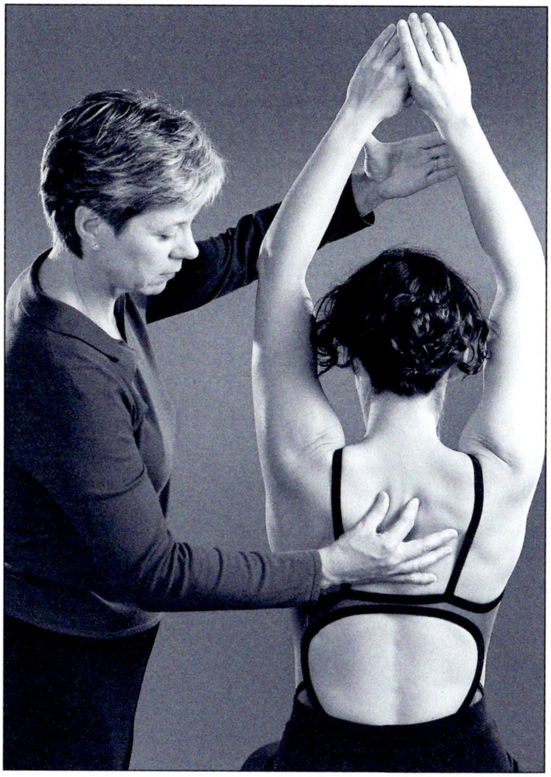

Figure 4.7 Functional movement testing – regional tests. Backward bending of the vertebromanubrial region occurs during bilateral elevation of the arms.

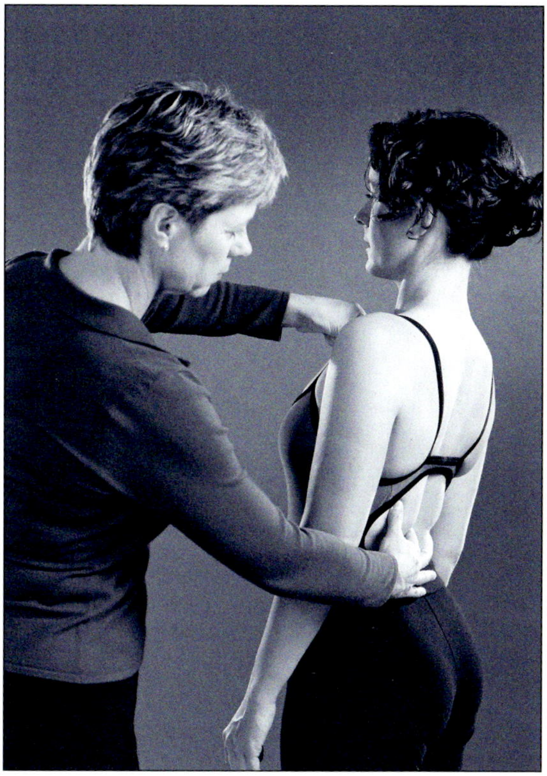

Figure 4.8 Functional movement testing – regional tests. Backward bending of the trunk.

should rest such that the medial border is parallel to the thoracic spine with the inferior angle approximated to the chest wall. Deviations of the spinous processes are common in the thoracic spine and often insignificant.

Deviation of the thorax from the three cardinal body planes is common (Figs. 4.2, 4.3, 4.4) and not necessarily associated with local symptoms. It can be caused by articular, neuromyofascial and/or emotional dysfunction.

Functional Movement Tests – Regional Tests

These tests examine the functional movements of the head and trunk. The quantity and pattern of available motion as well as the presence/location of provoked symptoms are noted.

Forward and backward bending

With the patient standing or sitting she is instructed to forward bend the head/trunk and the quantity and symmetry of motion is observed (Figs. 4.5, 4.6).

Backward bending of the vertebromanubrial region is achieved by asking the patient to elevate their arms bilaterally (Fig. 4.7). When examining backward bending of the vertebrosternal and vertebrochondral regions of the thorax (Fig. 4.8), it is critical to ensure that the region being examined is actually backward bending.

Neither rotation nor sideflexion should occur during forward nor backward bending (Willems et al 1996).

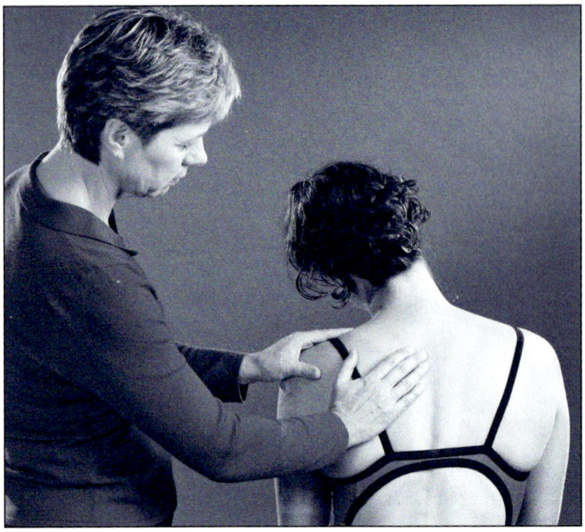

Figure 4.9 Functional movement testing – regional tests. Lateral bending of the head.

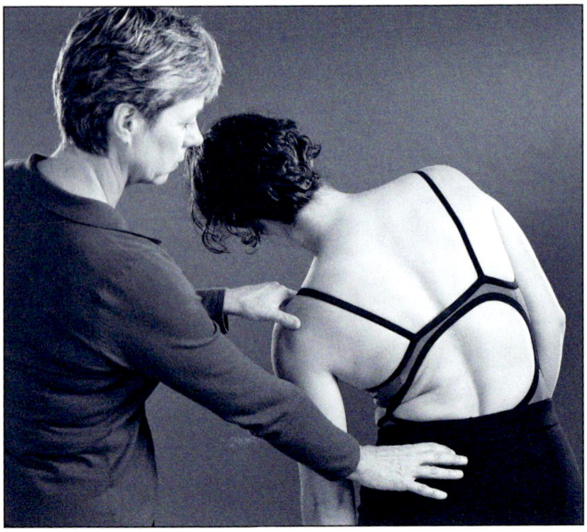

Figure 4.10 Functional movement testing – regional tests. Lateral bending of the trunk.

Lateral bending

With the patient standing or sitting she is instructed to laterally bend the head/trunk (Figs. 4.9, 4.10) to either side. The ability of the thorax to produce a smooth regional curve is noted. A flat region or a kink in the curve requires further specific mobility testing to determine the cause.

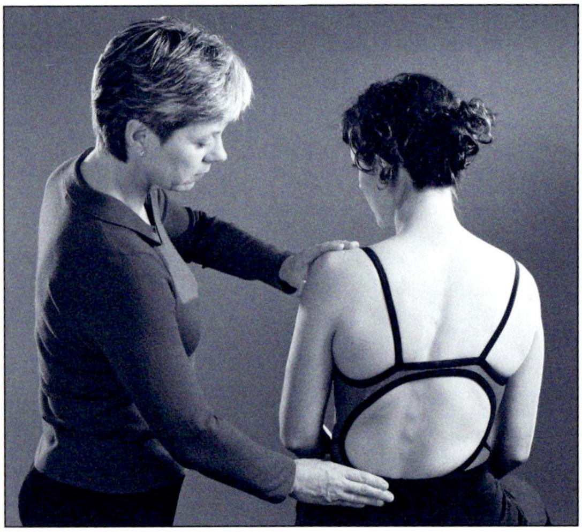

Figure 4.11 Functional movement testing – regional tests. Rotation of the trunk should produce a smooth S curve.

Axial rotation

With the patient standing or sitting she is instructed to rotate the head/trunk (Fig. 4.11) to either side. The ability of the thorax to produce a smooth regional S curve is noted. A lack of movement or a kink in the curve requires further specific mobility testing to determine the cause.

Respiration

With the patient standing or sitting she is instructed to take a deep breath in and a long breath out. Any asymmetry of chest expansion and release is noted and when present requires further specific mobility testing to determine the cause.

Functional Movement Tests – Segmental Tests

Forward bending

The following test is used to determine the osteokinematic function (active mobility) of two adjacent thoracic vertebrae during forward bending of the head/trunk. The transverse processes of two adjacent vertebrae are palpated with the index fingers and thumbs of both hands (Fig. 4.12a,b). The patient is instructed to forward bend the head/trunk and the quantity/symmetry of motion is noted during flexion of the thoracic segment. Both index fingers should travel an equal distance superiorly. When interpreting the mobility findings, the position of the joint at the beginning of the test should be correlated with the subsequent mobility noted, since alterations in joint mobility may merely be a reflection of an altered starting position. To determine the position of the superior vertebra, the dorsoventral relationship of the transverse processes to the coronal body plane is noted and compared with the level above and below. If the left transverse process of the superior vertebra is more dorsal than the left transverse process of the inferior vertebra then the segment is left rotated. If the left transverse process of the superior vertebra is less dorsal than the left transverse process of the inferior vertebra but more dorsal than the right transverse process of the superior vertebra, then the superior vertebra is relatively right rotated compared to the level below but left rotated when compared to the coronal body plane. This is a typical compensatory pattern seen when a superior segment is derotating or unwinding a primary rotation at a lower level.

The following test is used to determine the osteokinematic function (active mobility) of a rib relative to the vertebra of the same number during forward bending of the head/trunk. The transverse process is palpated with the thumb of one hand. The rib is palpated just lateral to the tubercle and medial to the angle with the thumb of the other hand (Fig. 4.13a,b). The index finger of this hand rests along the shaft of the rib. The patient is instructed to forward bend the head/trunk and the relative motion between the transverse process and the rib is noted.

In the mobile thorax, the rib continues to anteriorly rotate and the tubercle of the rib travels further superiorly than the transverse process at the end of the available range. In the stiffer thorax, the rib anteriorly rotates and the tubercle of the rib stops before full thoracic flexion is achieved such that the transverse process travels further superiorly than the rib at the end of the available range. When the relative mobility between the thoracic vertebra and the rib is the same, no motion is palpated between the vertebra and the rib during forward bending. To determine the patient's normal movement pattern it is critical to evaluate levels above, below and contralateral to the tested segment.

Backward bending

The following test is used to determine the osteokinematic function (active mobility) of two adjacent thoracic vertebrae during backward bending of the head/trunk. The transverse processes of two adjacent vertebrae are palpated with the index fingers and thumbs of both hands (Fig. 4.12a,b). The patient is instructed to backward

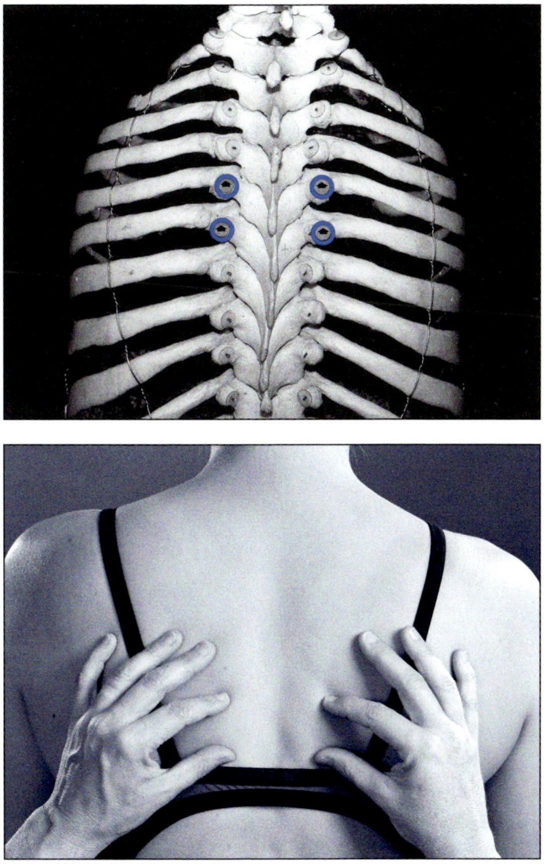

Figure 4.12a,b. Functional movement testing – segmental tests. Points of palpation for T5-6.

bend the trunk and the quantity/symmetry of motion is noted during extension of the thoracic segment. Backward bending of the upper thorax is achieved by asking the patient to elevate both arms. Both index fingers should travel an equal distance inferiorly. When interpreting the mobility findings, the position of the joint at the beginning of the test should be correlated with the subsequent mobility noted, since alterations in joint mobility may merely be a reflection of an altered starting position.

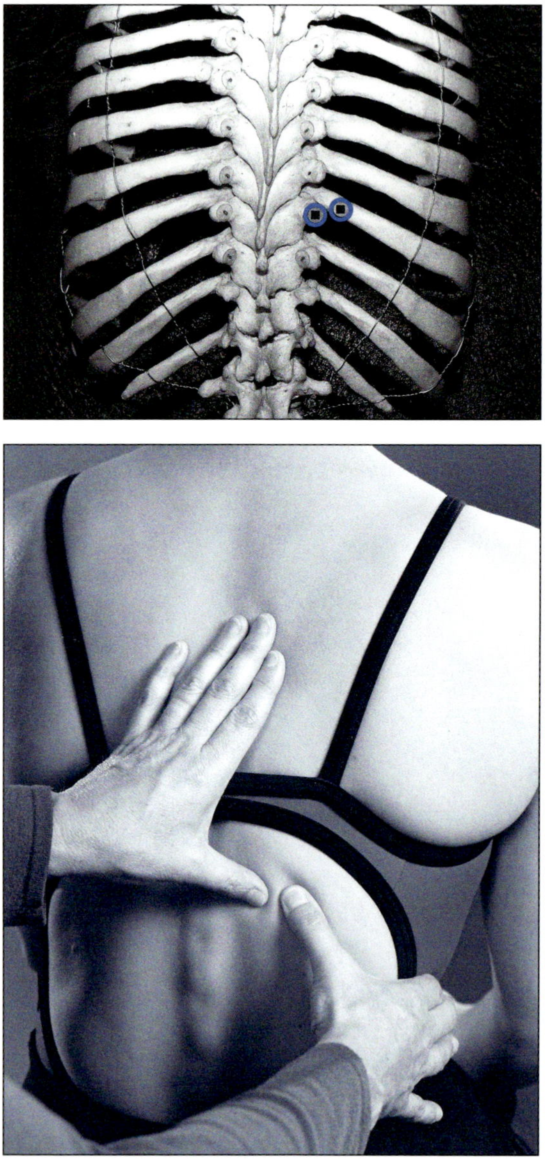

Figure 4.13a,b. Functional movement testing – segmental tests. Points of palpation for T9 – 9th rib.

The following test is used to determine the osteokinematic function (active mobility) of a rib and the vertebra of the same number during backward bending of the head/trunk. The transverse process is palpated with the thumb of one hand. The rib is palpated just lateral to the tubercle and medial to the angle with the thumb of the other hand (Fig. 4.13a,b). The index finger of this hand rests along the shaft of the rib. The patient is instructed to backward bend the trunk and the relative motion between the transverse process and the rib is noted. Backward bending of the upper thorax is achieved by asking the patient to elevate both arms.

In the mobile thorax, the rib continues to posteriorly rotate and the tubercle of the rib travels further inferiorly than the transverse process at the end of the available range. In the stiffer thorax, the rib posteriorly rotates and the tubercle of the rib stops before full thoracic extension is achieved such that the transverse process travels further inferiorly than the rib at the end of the available range. When the relative mobility between the thoracic vertebra and the rib is the same, no motion is palpated between the vertebra and the rib during backward bending. To determine the patient's normal movement pattern it is critical to evaluate levels above, below and contralateral to the tested segment.

Lateral bending

The following test is used to determine the osteokinematic function (active mobility) of two adjacent thoracic vertebrae during lateral bending of the head/trunk. The transverse processes of two adjacent vertebrae are palpated with the index fingers and thumbs of both hands. The patient is instructed to lateral bend the head/trunk and the quantity and direction of motion is noted. In the upper thorax, the superior thoracic vertebra should lateral bend and rotate to the same side such that the superior transverse process on the side of the concavity moves dorsally and inferiorly. Below T3, the superior thoracic vertebra should lateral bend in the pure coronal plane until the last few degrees of movement. At this point, the superior vertebra should rotate contralateral to the direction of the lateral bend.

Below T7, the direction of motion coupling depends on the apex of the curve (Chapter 3). The direction of rotation should be congruent with the levels above and below.

The following test is used to determine the osteokinematic function of a rib and the vertebra of the same number during lateral bending of the head/trunk. The transverse process is palpated with the thumb of one hand. The rib is palpated just lateral to the tubercle and medial to the angle with the thumb of the other hand. The index finger of this hand rests along the shaft of the rib. The patient is instructed to lateral bend the head/trunk and the relative motion between the transverse process and the rib is noted.

Rotation

The following test is used to determine the osteokinematic function of two adjacent thoracic vertebrae during rotation of the head/trunk. The transverse processes of two adjacent vertebrae are palpated with the index finger and thumb of both hands. The patient is instructed to rotate the head/trunk and the quantity and direction of motion is noted. In the upper thorax (vertebromanubrial) and the vertebrosternal regions, the superior thoracic vertebra should lateral bend and rotate to the same side such that the superior transverse process on the side of the concavity moves dorsally and inferiorly. Below T7, the direction of the conjunct lateral bend is variable. It may be either to the same side as the rotation or to the opposite side.

The following test is used to determine the osteokinematic function of a rib and the vertebra of the same number during rotation of the head/trunk. The transverse process is palpated with the thumb of one hand. The rib is palpated just lateral to the tubercle and medial to the angle with the thumb of the other hand. The index finger of this hand rests along the shaft of the rib. The patient is instructed to rotate the head/trunk and the relative motion between the transverse process and the rib is noted.

Respiration

The following test is used to determine the osteokinematic function of a rib relative to the vertebra of the same number during respiration. The transverse process is palpated with the thumb of one hand. The rib is palpated just lateral to the tubercle and medial to the angle with the thumb of the other hand. The index finger of this hand rests along the shaft of the rib. The patient is instructed to breathe in fully and the relative motion between the transverse process and the rib is noted. The patient is then instructed to breathe out fully and the relative motion between the transverse process and the rib is noted.

Articular Function – Form Closure

When a mobility abnormality is detected during the functional movement tests and localized to a segment with the active mobility tests, further examination is required to differentiate the role of the joints (form closure) and the muscles (force closure) in this movement aberration. The specific segmental tests of osteokinematic (passive physiological), arthrokinematic (passive accessory), and arthrokinetic (passive stability) function are used to differentiate the two.

Passive mobility tests of osteokinematic function

Passive physiological mobility tests are used to confirm the level of the abnormal movement pattern noted on active mobility testing. In addition,

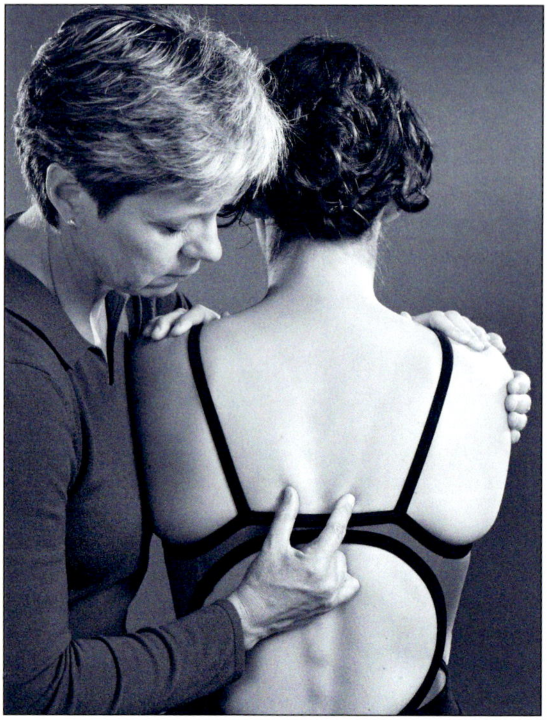

Figure 4.14 Articular function – form closure. Passive mobility tests of osteokinematic function.

the end feel of motion (analysis of the elastic zone of motion) is determined during these tests.

With the patient sitting and the arms crossed to the opposite shoulders for the vertebromanubrial and vertebrosternal regions, the transverse processes of the superior vertebra are palpated. In the thoracolumbar region, the interspinous space is palpated. The head/trunk is passively flexed, extended, laterally flexed and rotated (Fig. 4.14). The quantity of motion and the quality of the end feel is noted and compared to the levels above and below.

Passive mobility tests of arthrokinematic function

Zygapophyseal joints – Eg. T4-5 to test the superior glide of the right zygapophyseal joint. This test is used to determine the ability of the right inferior articular process of T4 to glide superiorly relative to the superior articular process of T5. With the patient prone and the thoracic spine in neutral, the inferior aspect of the left transverse process of T5 is palpated with one thumb. The other thumb palpates the inferior aspect of the right transverse process of T4. Fix T5 and apply a superoanterior glide to T4 (Figs. 4.15a,b).

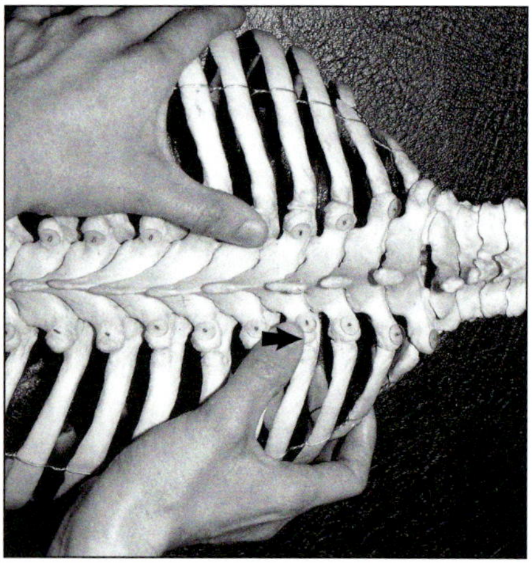

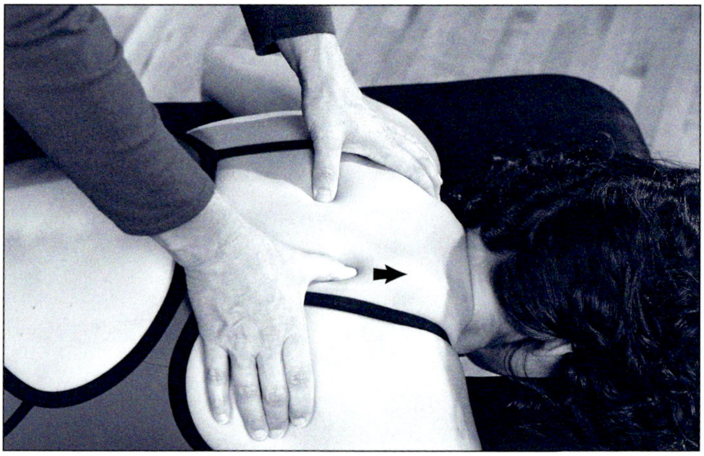

Figure 4.15a,b. Articular function – form closure. Passive mobility test of arthrokinematic function – points of palpation to test the superior glide of the right T4-5 zygapophyseal joint.

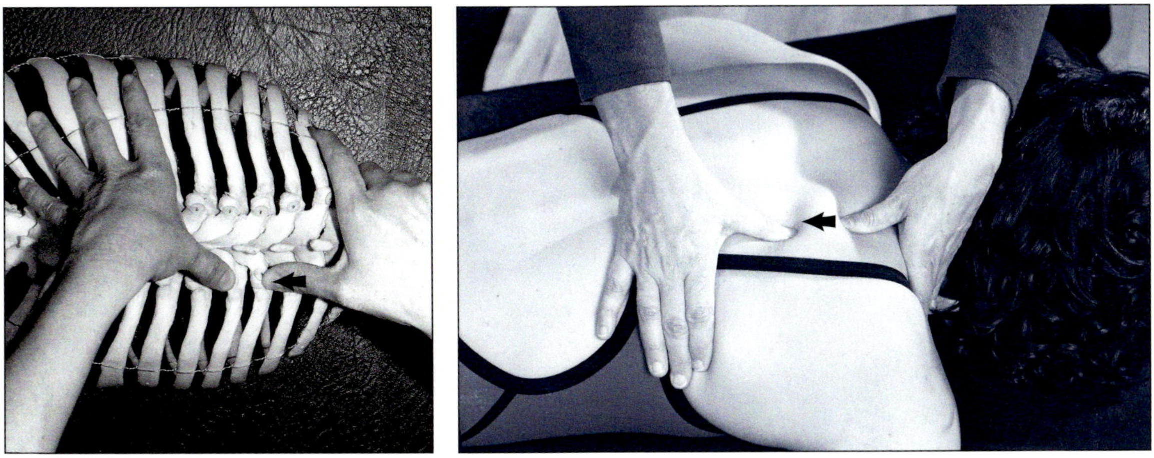

Figure 4.16a,b. Articular function – form closure. Passive mobility test of arthrokinematic function – points of palpation to test the inferior glide of the right T4-5 zygapophyseal joint.

The stiffness within the neutral zone and the quality of the elastic zone (end feel) is noted and compared to the contralateral side as well as to the levels above and below. This technique can be used for all thoracic segments.

Zygapophyseal joints – Eg. T4-5 to test the inferior glide of the right zygapophyseal joint. This test is used to determine the ability of the right inferior articular process of T4 to glide inferiorly relative to the superior articular process of T5. With the patient prone and the thoracic spine in neutral, the inferior aspect of the transverse process of T5 is palpated with one thumb. The other thumb palpates the superior aspect of the right transverse process of T4. Fix T5 and apply an inferior glide to T4 (Fig. 4.16a,b). The stiffness within the neutral zone and the quality of the elastic zone (end feel) is noted and compared to the contralateral side as well as to the levels above and below. This technique can be used for all thoracic segments.

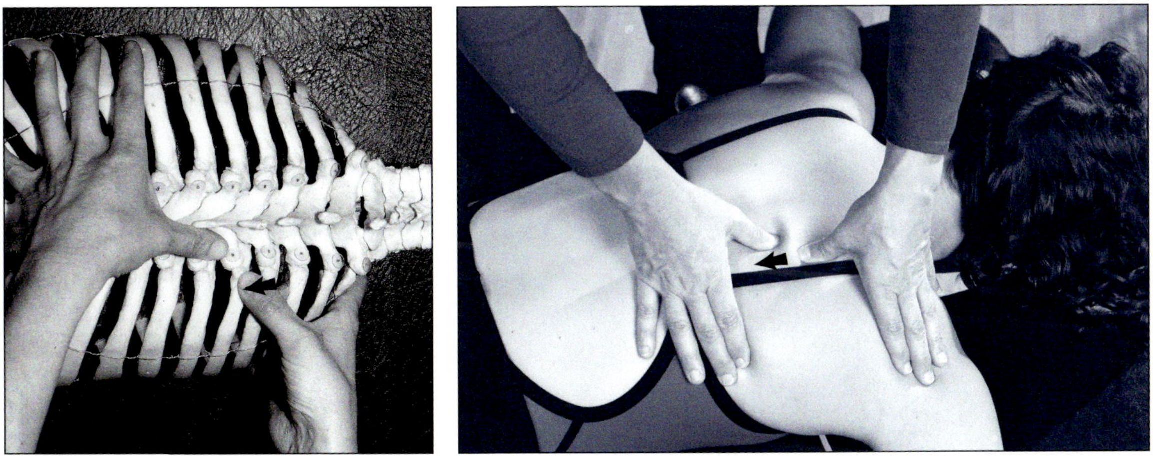

Figure 4.17a,b. Articular function – form closure. Passive mobility test of arthrokinematic function – points of palpation to test the inferior glide of the right fifth costotransverse joint.

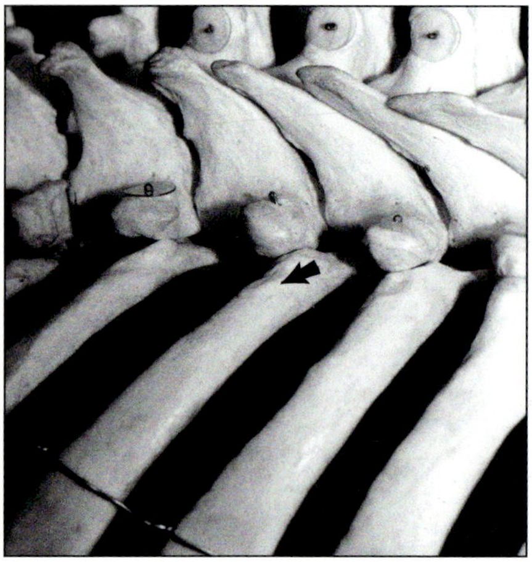
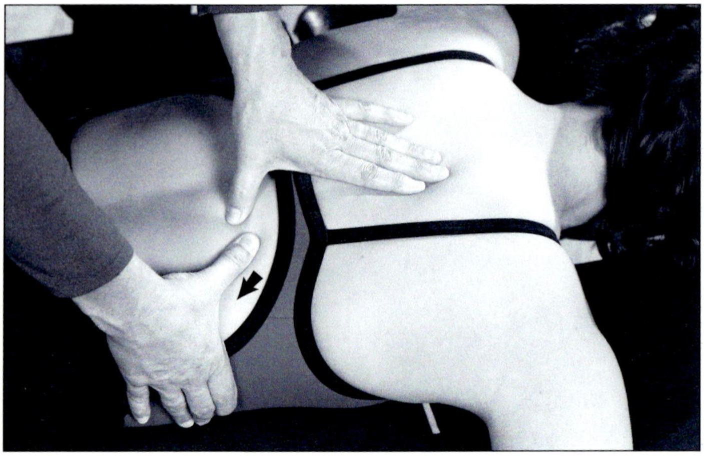

Figure 4.18a,b. Articular function – form closure. Passive mobility test of arthrokinematic function – points of palpation to test the anterolateroinferior (arrow) glide of the right 9th rib.

Costotransverse joints – Eg. To test the inferior glide of the right fifth rib at the costotransverse joint. This test is used to determine the ability of the right fifth rib to glide inferiorly relative to the transverse process of T5. With the patient prone and the thoracic spine in neutral, the inferior aspect of the right transverse process of T5 is palpated with one thumb. The other thumb palpates the superior aspect of the right fifth rib just lateral to the tubercle. Fix T5 and apply an inferior glide (allowing the conjunct posterior roll to occur) is applied to the fifth rib (Fig. 4.17a,b). The stiffness within the neutral zone and the quality of the elastic zone (end feel) is noted and compared to the contralateral side as well as to the levels above and below.

Between T7 and T10 the orientation of the costotransverse joint changes such that the direction of the glide is anterolateroinferior. The position of the right hand is modified to facilitate this change in joint direction such that the index finger

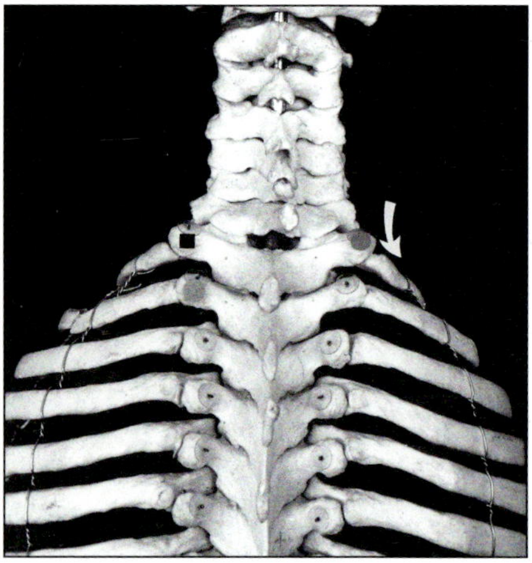
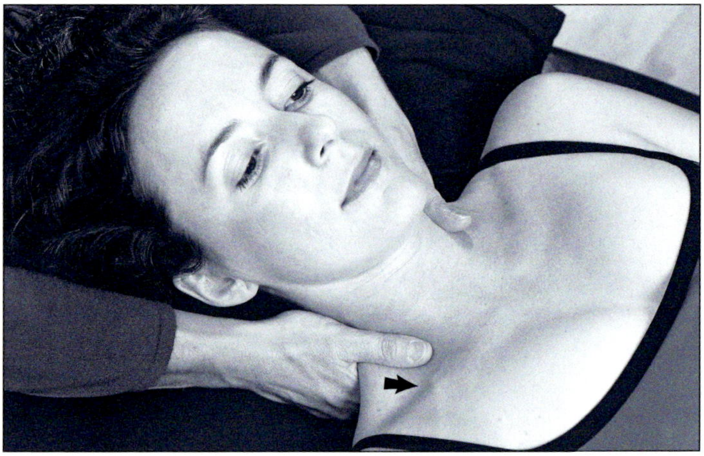

Figure 4.19a,b. Articular function – form closure. Passive mobility test of arthrokinematic function – points of palpation to test the inferior glide of the right 1st costotransverse joint.

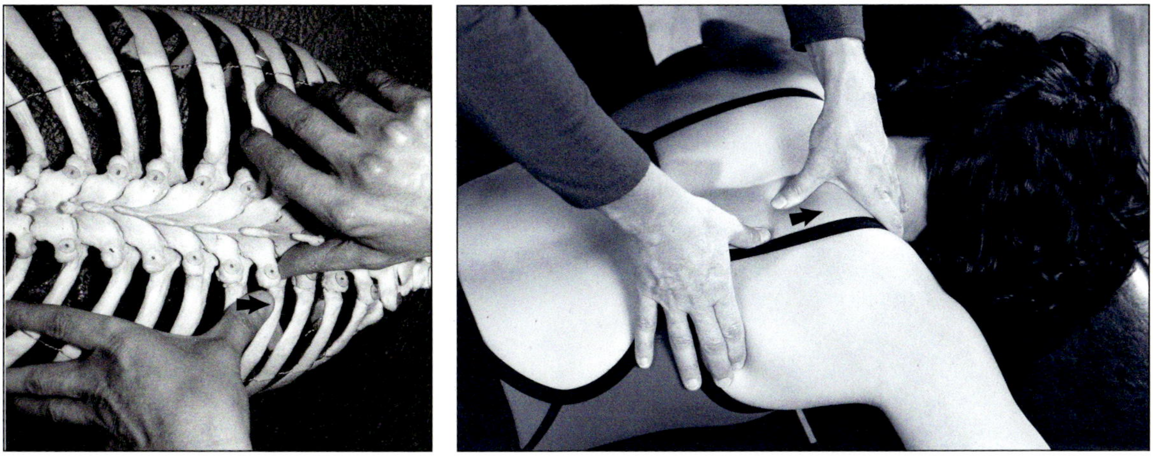

Figure 4.20a,b. Articular function – form closure. Passive mobility test of arthrokinematic function – points of palpation to test the superior glide of the right fifth costotransverse joint.

lies along the shaft of the rib and assists in gliding the rib in an anterolateroinferior direction (Fig. 4.18a,b).

Costotransverse joints – Eg. To test the inferior glide of the right first rib at the costotransverse joint. This test is used to determine the ability of the right first rib to glide inferiorly relative to the transverse process of T1. The patient lies supine with the head and neck comfortably supported on a pillow. With the lateral aspect of the MCP of the index finger of the left hand, the superior aspect of the left transverse process of T1 is palpated and fixed. With the lateral aspect of the MCP of the index finger of the right hand, the superior aspect of the right first rib is palpated just lateral to the costotransverse joint. The left hand fixes T1 and an inferior glide (allowing the conjunct posterior rotation to occur) is applied (Fig. 4.19a,b). The stiffness within the neutral zone and the quality of the elastic zone (end feel) is noted and compared to the contralateral side.

Costotransverse joints – Eg. To test the superior glide of the right fifth rib at the costotransverse joint. This test is used to determine the ability of the right fifth rib to glide superiorly relative to the transverse process of T5. With the patient prone and the thoracic spine in neutral, the superior aspect of the transverse process of T5 is palpated with one thumb. The other thumb palpates the inferior aspect of the right fifth rib just lateral to the tubercle. Fix T5 and apply a superior glide (allowing the conjunct anterior roll to occur) to the fifth rib (Fig. 4.20a,b). The stiffness within the neutral zone and the quality of the elastic zone (end feel) is noted and compared to the contralateral side as well as to the levels above and below.

Between T7 and T10 the orientation of the costotransverse joint changes such that the glide is posteromediosuperior. The position of the right hand is modified to facilitate this change in joint direction such that the index finger of the right hand lies along the shaft of the rib. The left hand fixes the transverse process while the right hand glides the rib posteromediosuperior (Fig. 4.21b). Alternately, the right hand can fix the rib while the transverse process is glided anterolateroinferior (Fig. 4.21a) thus producing a relative posteromediosuperior glide of the rib at the costotransverse joint.

Costotransverse joints – Eg. To test the superior glide of the right first rib at the costotransverse joint. This test is used to determine the ability of

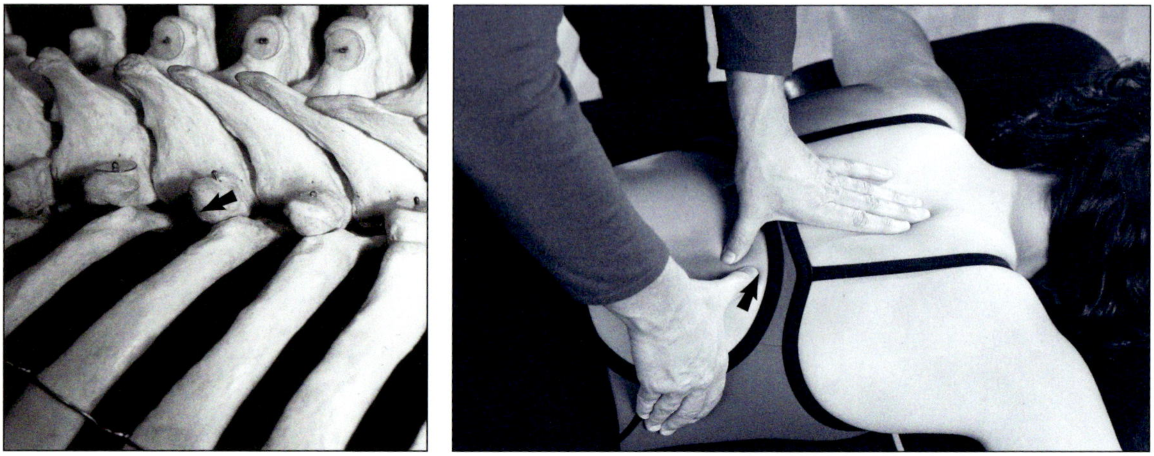

Figure 4.21a,b. Articular function – form closure. Passive mobility test of arthrokinematic function – points of palpation to test the posteromediosuperior glide of the right 9th rib. The T9 transverse process is glided anterolateroinferior.

the right first rib to glide superiorly relative to the transverse process of T1. The patient lies supine with the head and neck comfortably supported on a pillow. The superior aspect of the right transverse process of T1 is palpated with the right thumb. The index and middle fingers of the right hand palpate the inferior aspect of the right first rib. The right index and middle fingers fix the first rib and a posteroinferior glide is applied to the transverse process of T1 thus producing a relative superior glide of the first rib at the costotransverse joint (Fig. 4.22a,b). The stiffness within the neutral zone and the quality of the elastic zone (end feel) is noted and compared to the contralateral side.

Lateral translation – Eg. To test the ability of T5 and the right and left sixth ribs to glide transversely to the left on the T6 vertebra. This motion is necessary for full right rotation to occur. It requires the left sixth rib to glide posterolaterally relative to the left transverse process of T6 and

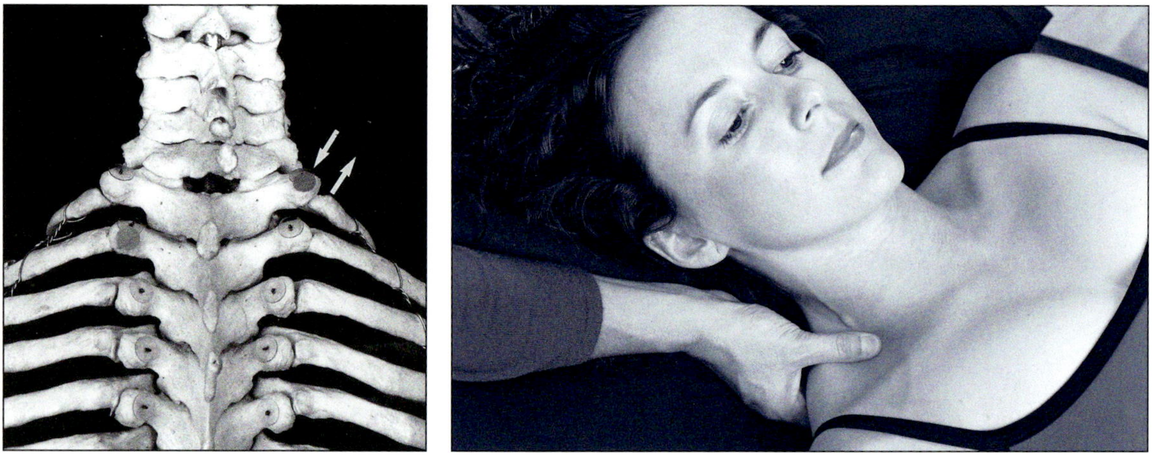

Figure 4.22a,b. Articular function – form closure. Passive mobility test of arthrokinematic function – points of palpation to test the superior glide of the right first costotransverse joint.

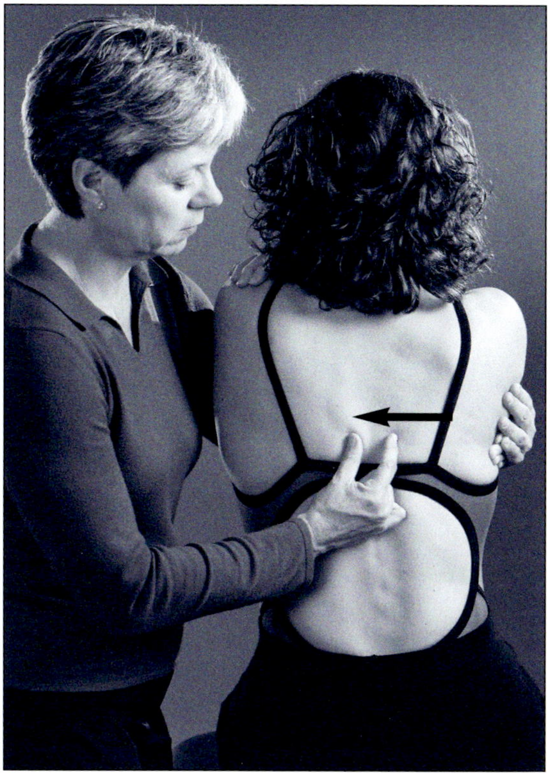

Figure 4.23. Articular function – form closure. Passive mobility test of arthrokinematic function – points of palpation to test lateral translation of T5 and the sixth ribs.

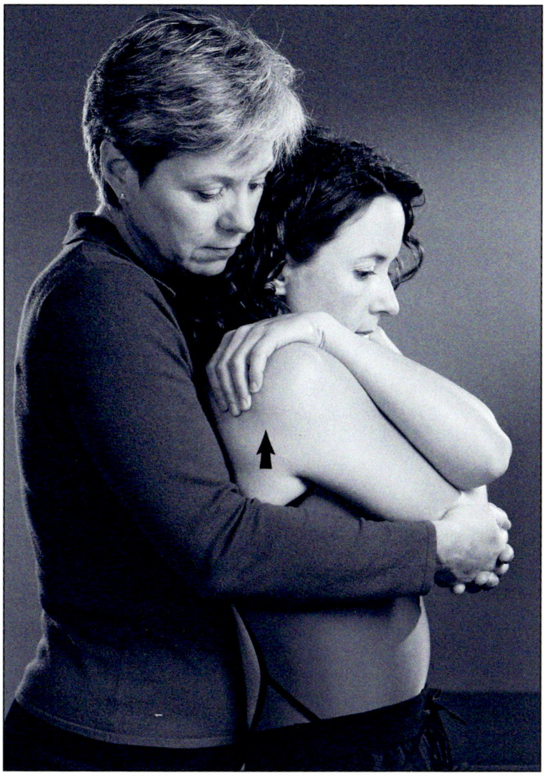

Figure 4.24. Articular function – form closure. Passive stability test of arthrokinetic function – traction midthorax.

the right sixth rib to glide anteromedially relative to the right transverse process of T6. The patient is sitting with the arms crossed to opposite shoulders. The therapist is standing at the patient's left side. With the left hand/arm, palpate the thorax such that the fifth finger of the left hand lies along the left sixth rib. With the right hand, palpate the transverse processes of T6. With the left hand/arm translate the T5 vertebra and the ribs PURELY to the left in the transverse plane (Fig. 4.23). The stiffness within the neutral zone and the quality of the elastic zone (end feel) is noted and compared to the contralateral side as well as to the levels above and below.

Passive stability tests of arthrokinetic function

Vertical (traction/compression). This test stresses the anatomical structures which resist vertical forces. The patient is sitting with the arms crossed to opposite shoulders such that the arm closest to the chest grasps the scapula. The other arm rests on top of the contralateral shoulder. The thoracic spine is in neutral. Traction is applied to the middle and lower thorax by applying a vertical force through the patient's crossed arms (Fig. 4.24). Traction is applied to the upper thorax by applying a vertical force through the cranium. Compression is applied to the middle and lower thorax by applying a vertical force through the top of the patient's shoulders (Fig. 4.25).

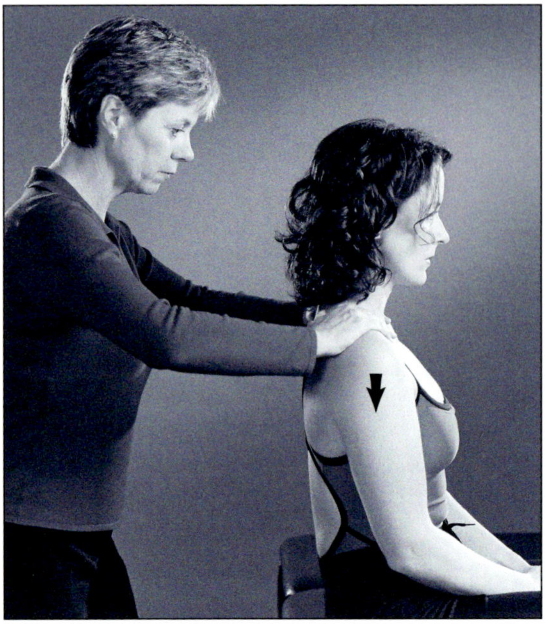

Figure 4.25. Articular function – form closure. Passive stability test of arthrokinetic function – compression midthorax.

Compression is applied to the upper thorax by applying a vertical force through the cranium. A positive response is the reproduction of the patient's pain as opposed to a sense of increased osteoarticular motion.

Anterior translation – spinal. This test stresses the anatomical structures that resist anterior translation of a segmental spinal unit. With the patient prone lying, the transverse processes of the inferior vertebra are fixed. With the other hand, the transverse processes of the superior vertebra are palpated. An posteroanterior force is applied through the superior vertebra while fixing the inferior vertebra (Fig. 4.26a,b). The stiffness within the neutral zone and the quality of the elastic zone (end feel) is noted and compared to the levels above and below. The findings from this test should be correlated with those of the posterior translation test to determine the level of the instability. Excessive anterior translation of the T4 vertebra could be due to either an anterior instability of T4-5 or a posterior instability of T3-4.

Posterior translation – spinal. This test stresses the anatomical structures that resist posterior translation of a segmental spinal unit. The patient is sitting with the arms crossed to opposite shoulders. The thorax is stabilized with one hand/arm under/over (depending on the level) the patient's crossed arms. The transverse processes of the inferior vertebra are fixed with the dorsal hand. Stability is tested by applying an anteroposterior force to the superior vertebra through the thorax

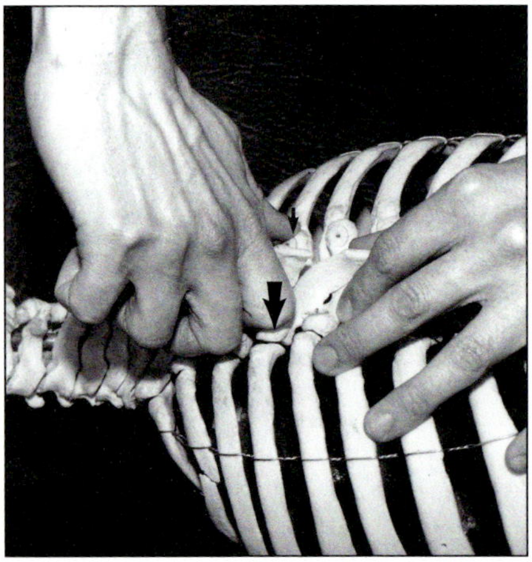

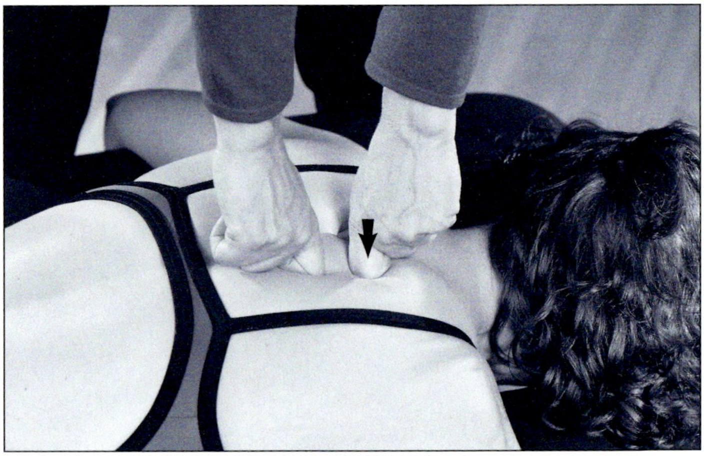

Figure 4.26a,b. Articular function – form closure. Passive stability test for arthrokinetic function – points of palpation to test anterior translation (spinal).

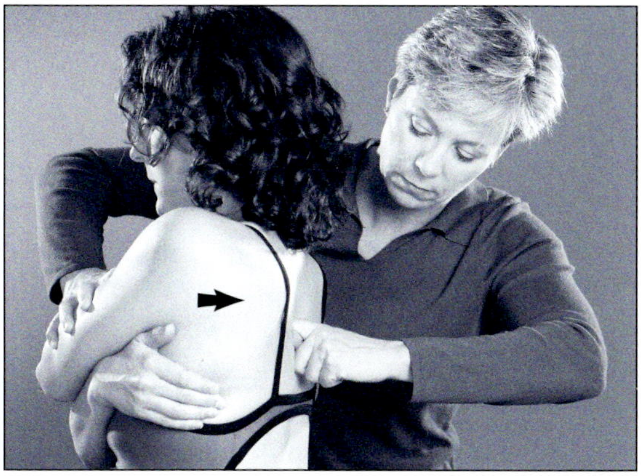

Figure 4.27. Articular function – form closure. Passive stability test for arthrokinetic function – points of palpation to test posterior translation (spinal).

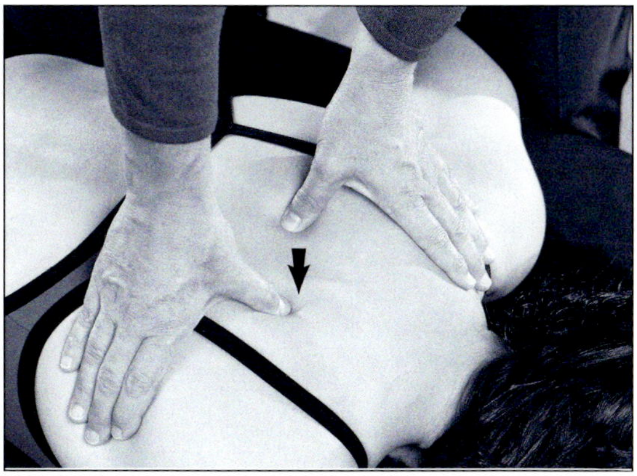

Figure 4.28. Articular function – form closure. Passive stability test for arthrokinetic function – points of palpation to test left rotation (spinal).

while fixing the inferior vertebra (Fig. 4.27). The stiffness within the neutral zone and the quality of the elastic zone (end feel) is noted and compared to the levels above and below. The findings from this test should be correlated with those of the anterior translation test to determine the level of the instability.

Transverse rotation – spinal. This test stresses the anatomical structures which resist rotation of a segmental spinal unit. With the patient prone lying, the transverse process of the superior vertebra is palpated. With the other hand, the contralateral transverse process of the inferior vertebra is fixed. A transverse plane rotation force is applied through the superior vertebra by applying a unilateral posteroanterior pressure while fixing the inferior vertebra (Fig. 4.28). The stiffness within the neutral zone and the quality of the elastic zone (end feel) is noted and compared to the contralateral side and the levels above and below.

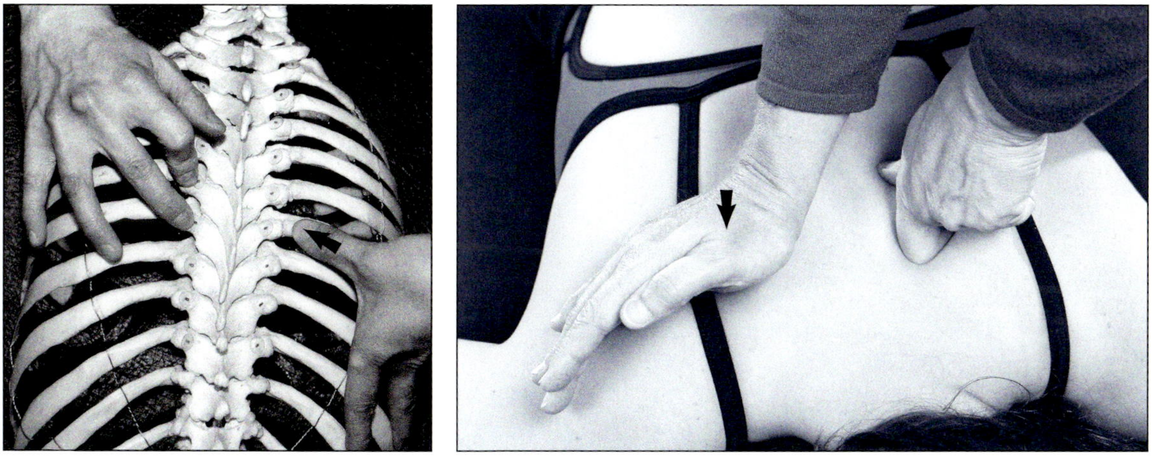

Figure 4.29a,b. Articular function – form closure. Passive stability test for arthrokinetic function – points of palpation to test anterior translation (posterior costal).

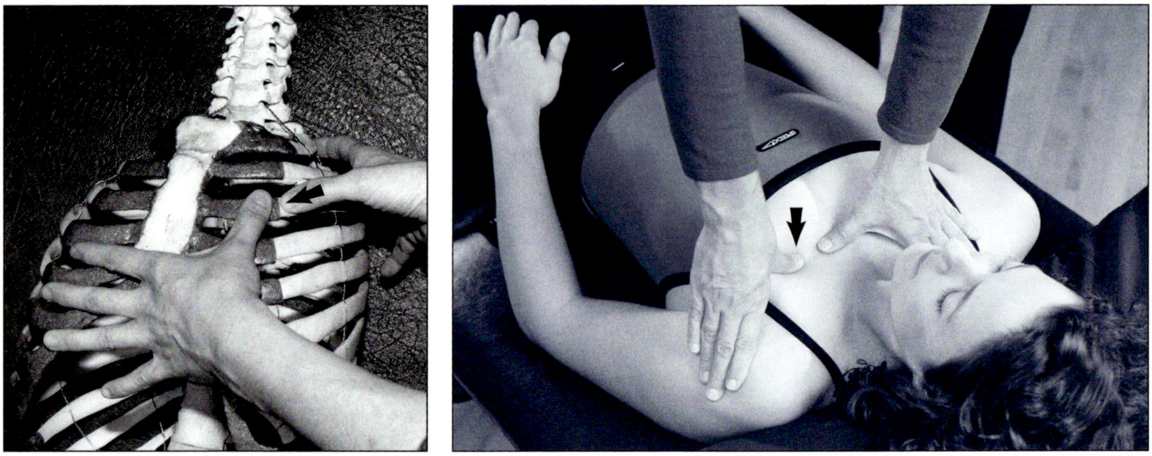

Figure 4.30a,b. Articular function – form closure. Passive stability test for arthrokinetic function – points of palpation to test anteroposterior translation (anterior costochondral).

Anterior translation – posterior costal. This test stresses the anatomical structures which resist anterior translation of the posterior aspect of the rib relative to the thoracic vertebrae to which it attaches (Lowcock 1990). With the patient prone lying, the contralateral transverse processes of the thoracic vertebrae to which the rib is attached are palpated. For example, when testing the right fifth rib the left transverse processes of T5 and T4 are palpated. With the other hand, the rib is palpated just lateral to the tubercle (Fig. 4.29). A posteroanterior force is applied to the rib while fixing the thoracic vertebrae. The stiffness within the neutral zone and the quality of the elastic zone (end feel) is noted and compared to the contralateral side.

Anterior/Posterior translation – anterior costal. This test stresses the anatomical structures which resist translation of the costocartilage relative to the sternum; and the rib relative to the costocartilage. When the sternocostal and/or costochondral joints have been separated, a gap and a step can be palpated at the joint line. The positional findings are noted prior to stressing the joint. With one thumb, the anterior aspect of the sternum/costocartilage is palpated. With the other thumb, the anterior aspect of the costocartilage/rib is palpated. An anteroposterior/posteroanterior force is applied to the costocartilage/rib (Fig. 4.30). The stiffness the neutral zone and the quality of the elastic zone (end feel) is noted and compared to the contralateral side.

Lateral translation. This test stresses the anatomical structures which resist horizontal translation between two adjacent vertebrae when the ribs between them are fixed. This test is used between the segments T3-4 and T10-11. The primary structure being tested is the intervertebral disc. To test the T5-6 segment, the patient is sitting with the arms crossed to opposite shoulders. With the left hand/arm, the thorax is palpated such that the fifth finger of the left hand lies along the fifth rib. With the right hand, the left sixth rib is compressed centrally towards the costovertebral joint (Fig. 4.31). The T5 vertebra is translated through the thorax PURELY to the left in the transverse plane. When the rib is fixed against the vertebral body there should be very little, if any, lateral translation between two thoracic vertebrae.

Neuromyofascial Function – Force Closure and Motor Control

Palpation of the segmental local stabilizers

The local stabilizers for the thorax include the deep fibers of multifidus, rotatores breves, levator costarum and the intercostals. To date, there has been no research to validate this classification and this hypothesis comes from knowledge gained from the research of the lumbopelvic region (see Chapter 2). Clinically, it has been noted that atrophy of these deep small muscles occurs subsequent to injury to the thorax. Like the lumbar spine, the affect appears to be segmental. The muscles are palpated with the patient prone lying, head in neutral and arms resting comfortably over the sides of the table. The 'gutter' between the spinous process and the transverse process is palpated (Fig. 4.32). Press firmly, but gently, into the tissue and note the quality of the tissue (firmness) and the size of the muscle. Compare the firmness/size to the contralateral side and to levels above and below.

Prone Arm Lift

This test was initially proposed by Linda-Joy Lee, working together with Bill Lyons in the development of tests for evaluating dynamic stability of the thorax. It evolved from the Active Straight Leg Raise Test (ASLR) (Mens et al 1997, 1999, 2001); a validated test of load transfer/stability of the lumbopelvic region. The prone patient is asked to lift their arm off of the table (only a few degrees of lift is necessary) (Fig. 4.33) and to note any difference in the effort required to lift the left or right arm (does one arm seem heavier or harder to lift). The strategy used to stabilize the thorax during this task is observed. The arm should flex at the glenohumeral joint, the scapula should remain upwardly rotated and stable against the chest wall, the thorax should not rotate, sidebend, flex, extend or translate. If the arm is elevated to the end of its available range then the thorax will move; this is a normal biomechanical consequence. Therefore, when interpreting the findings from this test it is important to observe what happens in the thorax during the moment the arm begins to lift. The provocation of any pain is also noted at this time. The thorax is then compressed passively (Fig. 4.34) by approximating the ribs (noted to be moving during the first part

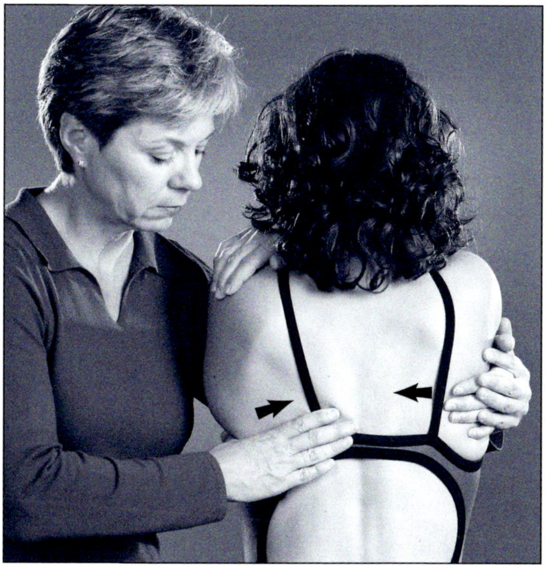

Figure 4.31. Articular function – form closure. Passive stability test for arthrokinetic function – T5-6 right lateral translation stability test.

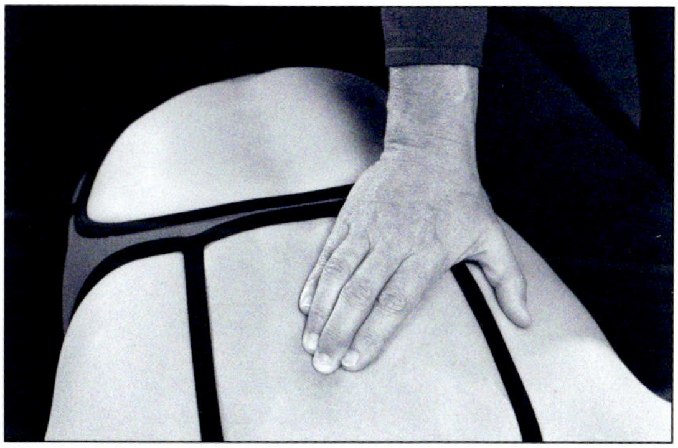

Figure 4.32 Neuromyofascial Function – force closure and motor control. Palpation of the segmental local stabilizers.

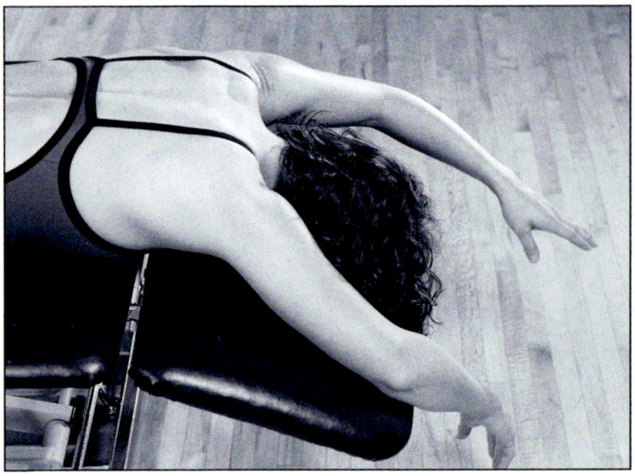

Figure 4.33 The Prone Arm Lift is used to evaluate dynamic stability of the thorax during loading.

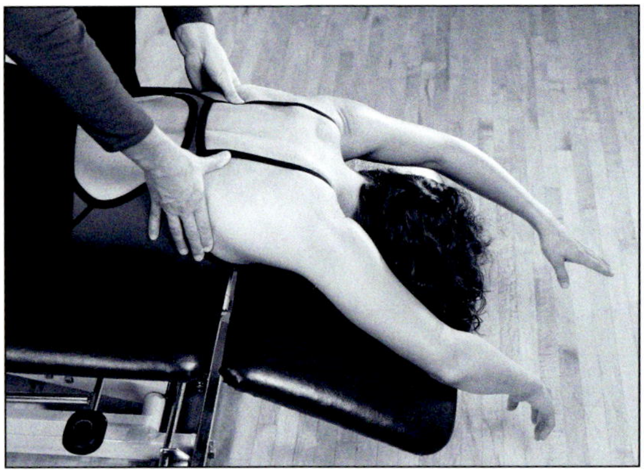

Figure 4.34 The impact of manual compression of the thorax through the rib cage is noted on both pain provocation and effort to lift the arm.

of this test) towards the midline either anteriorly or posteriorly. The Prone Arm Lift is repeated and any change in effort and/or pain is noted.

Test for the integrity of the active force closure mechanism

When the active force closure mechanism is effective, co-contraction of the muscles of the local muscle system should compress the thoracic segment thereby reducing the neutral zone for both horizontal and vertical translation. This has been verified for the SIJ (Richardson et al 2002). To test the status of the active force closure mechanism, the patient is first instructed to recruit the local muscle system (see Chapter 7). This instruction may take a few sessions to master. Once the patient is able to sustain a tonic co-contraction of the local muscle system, the effect of this contraction on the neutral zone is assessed by repeating the form closure tests for anteroposterior and/or lateral translation (see above). The stiffness should increase and no relative intersegmental or vertebrocostal motion should be felt. This means that an adequate amount of compression of the thorax has occurred and the force closure mechanism is effective. If the neutral zone motion remains "excessive" compared to the adjacent levels and the local muscle system is contracting appropriately, then the active force closure mechanism is ineffective for controlling shear. This is a poor prognostic sign for successful rehabilitation with exercise.

Neural Conduction and Mobility

These tests examine the conductivity of the motor and sensory nerves as well as the mobility of the dura and the intercostal nerves in the spinal canal and intervertebral foramen. The sensory function of the intercostal nerves is examined by testing skin sensation in the intercostal spaces. Altered sensation is not uncommon although rarely reported as a primary complaint. Hyperaesthesia can be one of the first signs of neurological interference and tends to occur long before sensation becomes reduced (hypoaesthesia).

The motor function of the intercostal nerves is examined by observing and palpating the intercostal muscles. Segmental facilitation leads to hypertonicity of the intercostal muscle and the increased tone can be palpated along the intercostal space. The tone is often associated with tender points within the muscle. Reduced motor function of the intercostal nerves causes atrophy of the intercostal muscles.

Reflex tests are used to detect spinal cord or upper motor neuron lesions. The plantar response test and the test for clonus should be done on every patient presenting with pain in the thorax.

The mobility tests for the neural and dural tissue (Butler 2000) include the slump test and variations thereof. The mobility of the intraspinal tissues can be tested by fully lengthening the dural/neural system. This is achieved by having the seated patient fully flex the head and neck, slump the thoracolumbar spine and extend the knee with the ankle dorsiflexed. The dura is released by then having the patient extend the head and neck. The change in symptom response is noted. If the thoracic pain is brought on by full slump and relieved with extension of the head and neck, involvement of the dura is suggested (Butler 2000).

The intercostal nerves can be further tensed by having the 'slumped' patient twist the thorax to the left and right. Often, the patient will present with a normal movement pattern when rotation occurs in a position of relative neural relaxation and an abnormal movement pattern (segmental kink in the thoracic curve) when the rotation occurs in a position of relative neural tension. It is interesting to postulate on the etiology of the 'apparent segmental dysfunction' in this situation and unless the nervous system is addressed, the symptoms persist regardless of the articular and myofascial treatments employed. The emphasis of this text is on the assessment and treatment of articular and myofascial dysfunction and the reader is referred to Butler's work on this subject for further review.

Adjunctive Tests

While X-rays exclude serious bone disease and significant mechanical defects, they rarely provide guidance for physical therapy. Asymmetry is the rule in the thorax and deviation of the spinous processes is to be expected. For the physical therapist, the primary reason for obtaining the results of any adjunctive imaging tests is to rule out serious pathology and to identify anatomical anomalies which may influence the interpretation of mobility analysis. The findings noted on adjunctive testing of the thorax must be correlated with the findings noted on clinical examination if the significance is to be understood.

The Integrated Model of Function

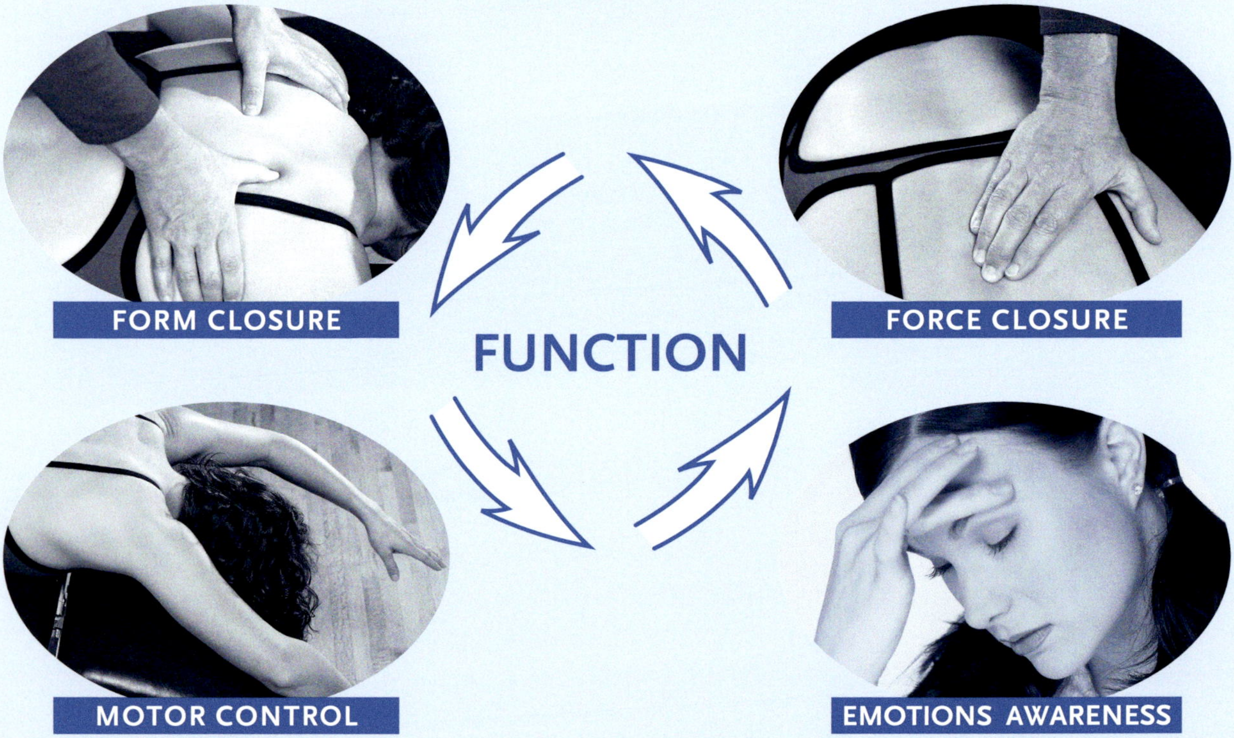

5

CLASSIFYING THE THORACIC DYSFUNCTION

Functionally, motion of the thorax can become restricted or poorly controlled due to either excessive or insufficient articular compression. In keeping with the integrated model, the causes for the thoracic impairment can be due to dysfunction of

- **form closure (structure),**
- **force closure (forces produced by myofascial action/inaction) and**
- **motor control (specific timing of muscle action/inaction during loading)**

In addition, force closure and motor control can be impacted by the emotional state of the patient.

INTEGRATED MODEL OF FUNCTION CLASSIFICATION

Functionally, motion of the thorax can become restricted or poorly controlled due to either excessive or insufficient articular compression. In keeping with the integrated model, the causes for the thoracic impairment can be due to dysfunction of:

- form closure (structure),
- force closure (forces produced by myofascial action/inaction) and
- motor control (specific timing of muscle action/inaction during loading)

In addition, force closure and motor control can be impacted by the emotional state of the patient.

Excessive Articular Compression

Excessive articular compression can result from articular pathology (ankylosing spondylitis or diffuse idiopathic skeletal hyperostosis (DISH)), fibrosis of the articular capsule or overactivation of muscles. The fused joints cannot be mobilized whereas the fibrosed joints require specific mobilization. When the excessive compression is secondary to muscle imbalance, appropriate motor control training which emphasizes optimal stabilization strategies (see Chapter 7) will be required.

Excessive Articular Compression with an Underlying Instability

When a force is applied to the joint sufficient to attenuate the articular ligaments, the muscles will respond to prevent dislocation and further trauma to the joint. The resulting spasm fixes the joint in an abnormal resting position and marked asymmetry of the bones is present. This is an unstable joint under excessive compression. Treatment usually requires a manipulation to distract the joint. These techniques will reduce the articular compression and restore the resting position of the bones. Repeat analysis of the form closure tests (passive tests for arthrokinematic function, also known as joint play) will now reveal a decrease in stiffness compared to the opposite side. Restoration of the force closure mechanism through an appropriate exercise program must follow. This is an impairment of both form and force closure in that the relationship between the articular surfaces has been disturbed and the muscle response is excessive.

Treatment of this individual which focuses on exercise without first addressing the "posture", "position", alignment" of the thorax, tends to be ineffective and commonly increases symptoms. Conversely, if treatment only includes manual therapy (mobilization, manipulation or muscle energy) for correction of "posture", "position", "alignment", relief tends to be temporary and dependence on the health care practitioner providing the manual correction is common. This impairment requires a combination of manual therapy, exercise and education for a successful outcome.

Insufficient Articular Compression

Insufficient articular compression occurs when there is either

- inadequate or inappropriate motor control during movement and loading or
- overstretching of the ligaments which restrain the end range of the articular motion.

Treatment requires the restoration of the active force closure mechanism (see Chapter 7) with specific exercises that initially isolate the muscles required for stabilization followed by a program that addresses motor control.

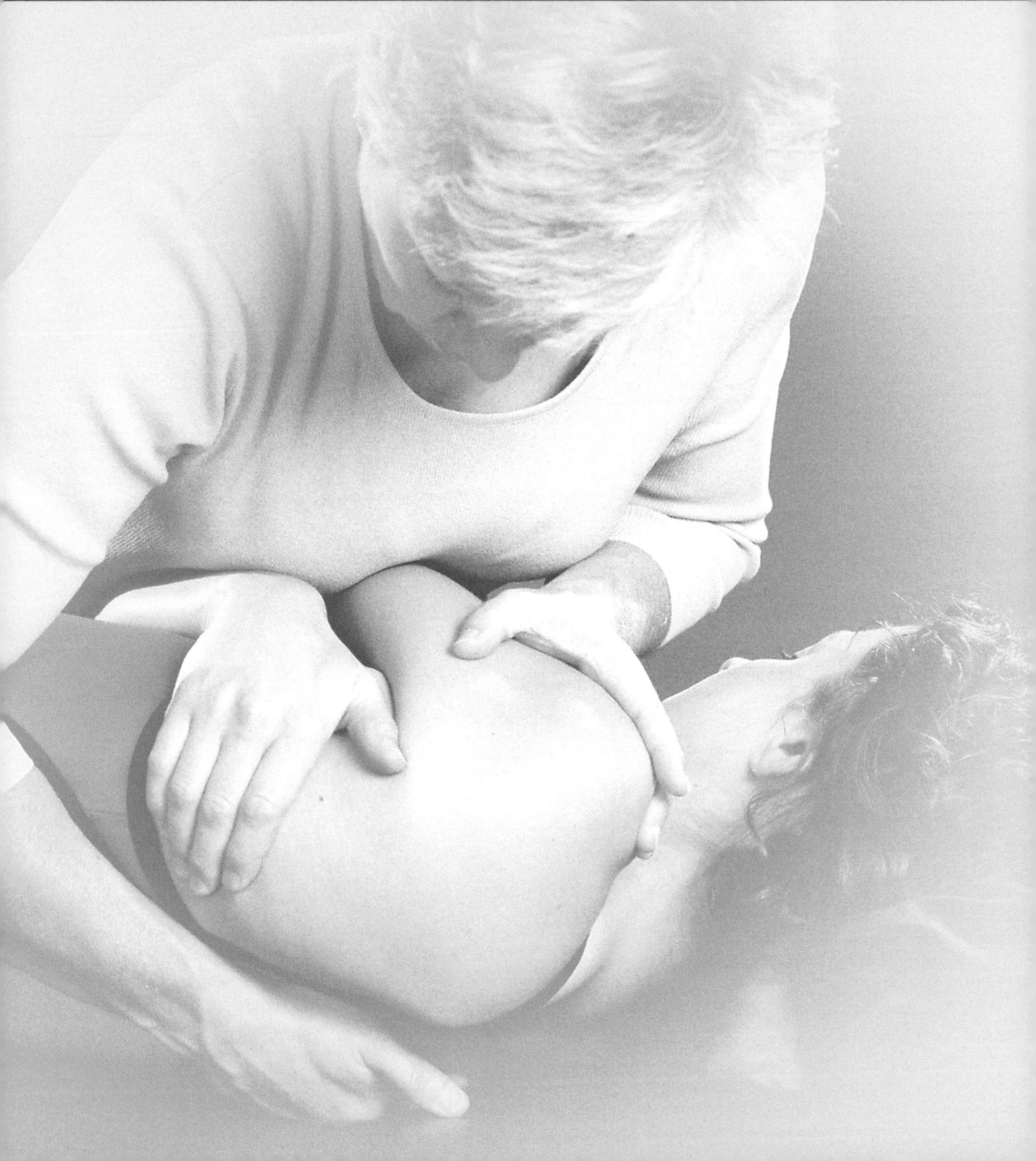

6

RESTORING FORM CLOSURE OF THE THORAX

This chapter will describe the clinical findings of excessive articular compression. Specific articular mobilization techniques for the stiff joint, "muscle release/decompression" techniques for the "compressed" joint and manipulation techniques for the fixated joint will be described.

The reader is referred to the CD-ROM which accompanies this text to view short video clips of these techniques.

This chapter will describe the clinical findings of excessive articular compression secondary to either

- fibrosis of the zygapophyseal or costotransverse joint (stiff joint) or
- overactivation of the segmental muscles which are compressing the zygapophyseal or constotransverse joint (compressed joint) or
- a costotransverse joint fixation or a fixation of the entire thoracic ring (excessive articular compression with an underlying instability).

Specific articular mobilization techniques for the stiff joint, 'muscle release/decompression' techniques for the 'compressed' joint and manipulation techniques for the fixated joint will be described. The reader is referred to the CD-ROM which accompanies this text to view short video clips of these techniques.

Although this chapter focuses mainly on excessive compression through the posterior joints of the thorax, some mention should be made of thoracic intervetebral disc herniations. Magnetic resonance imaging (MRI) has increased the frequency of this diagnosis. Brown et al (1992) confirmed that thoracic disc herniations produce anterior chest pain (67%). Other symptoms included lower extremity dysaesthesia and weakness (20%), interscapular pain (8%) and epigastric pain (4%). "The degree of herniation was characterized as mild, moderate, or severe. A mild herniation consisted of only minimal dural indentation. Moderate herniation created limited cord pressure with no significant deformation. Severe herniations resulted in free fragments or evidence of cord compression manifested by indentation or flattening of the cord." The highest incidence according to level was T7-8, the second highest was T6-7 and T9-10. The irritability of the painful tissue dictates the intensity of the pain, the amount of radiation, the degree of physical activity which tends to aggravate it and the amount of rest required to relieve it. The intervertebral disc herniation causes excessive compression of the thorax due to secondary muscle spasm/hypertonicity. Specific and/or regional distraction techniques as well as muscle release/decompression techniques are often helpful for relieving pain. In addition, postural education, taping for support and time complete the management of this condition.

EXCESSIVE ARTICULAR COMPRESSION – STIFF JOINT

Fibrosis of the zygapophyseal and/or costotransverse joint is usually related to a traumatic event although habitually sustained postures can also lead to multisegmental joint stiffness. In the case of segmental joint stiffness, the location of pain may be on the ipsilateral or contralateral side of the stiff joint and may radiate around or through to the anterior aspect of the chest. An acute zygapophyseal joint sprain tends to produce localized pain over the involved joint. A chronic restriction of either the zygapophyseal or costovertebral joint tends to produce symptoms removed from the source (contralateral side of the thorax or at levels above or below). The joints of the thorax tend to refer pain around the chest whereas the intervertebral disc tends to refer pain through the chest.

The stiff, fibrotic joint will present with the following objective findings.

1. **Postural analysis.**
   The impact of a stiff joint on an individual's posture depends on whether the fibrosis is confined to a single segment or spans multiple segments. A segmental, fibrotic joint may not reveal itself through postural analysis. Alternately, it may stand out as a segmental rotation in the

midst of an otherwise normal curve. Multisegmental stiffness tends to alter the primary thoracic curve and can be exaggerated (kyphosis), reduced (lordosis) or twisted (rotoscoliosis).

2. **Functional movement tests and active mobility tests of osteokinematic function.**
   Both the segmental stiff joint and the multisegmental stiff region present with a consistent pattern of asymmetric motion. If the restriction is bilateral, then a symmetric reduction of movement is noted compared to levels above and below. The unilaterally restricted zygapophyseal joint presents with an ipsilateral restriction pattern (sideflexion and rotation restricted to the same side). The unilaterally restricted costotransverse joint presents with a contralateral restriction pattern (sideflexion and rotation restricted to opposite sides).

3. **Articular function – form closure.**
   Both the segmental stiff joint and the multisegmental stiff region present with a consistent pattern of restriction on segmental passive mobility testing. Increased stiffness in the neutral zone and a harder end feel in the elastic zone are noted on passive tests for arthrokinematic function. The stiff joint has a solid stop which does not vary with the speed of the test.

4. **Neuromyofascial function – force closure and motor control.**
   The Prone Am Lift test may reveal poor thoracic position control segmentally and/or multisegmentally.

5. **Neural conduction and mobility.**
   Conduction is normal and neural/dural mobility may or may not be restricted.

6. **Adjunctive tests.**
   X-rays are rarely helpful; they may reveal a rotoscoliotic or kypholordotic curve which is also evident on postural analysis.

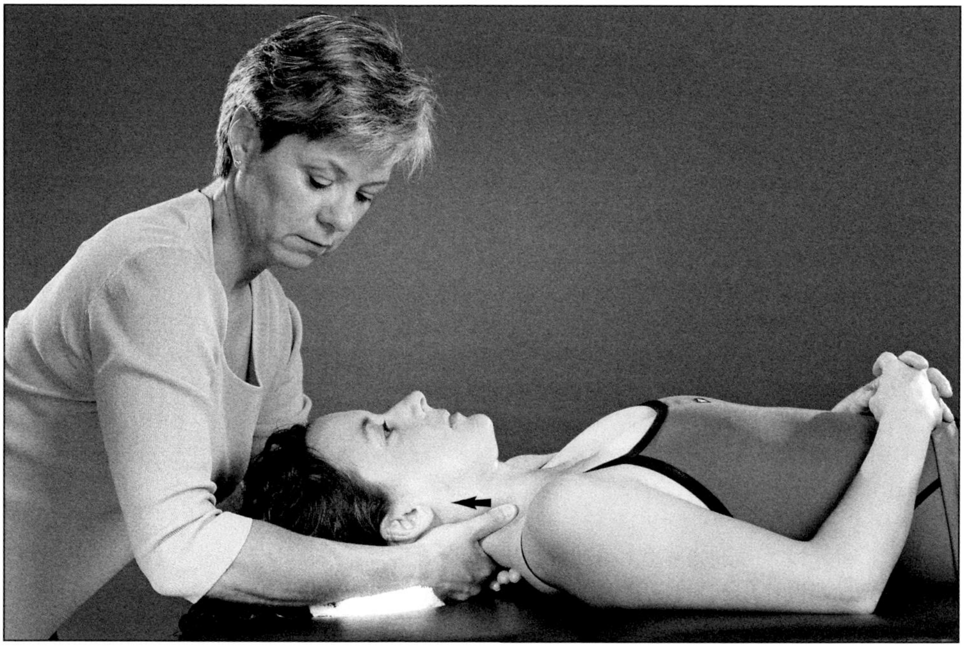

Figure 6.1. Bilateral flexion restriction – vertebromanubrial region. Longitudinal traction – supine.

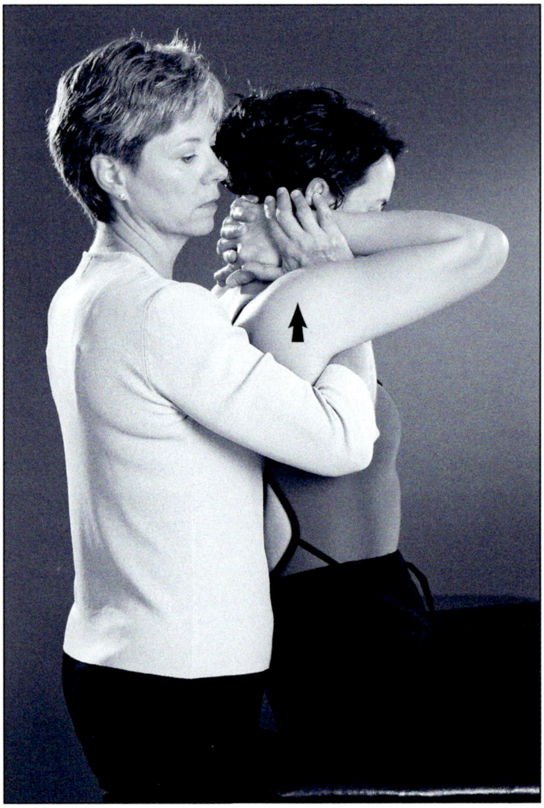

Figure 6.2. – Bilateral flexion restriction – vertebromanubrial region. Longitudinal traction – sitting.

The next section of this chapter will describe/illustrate specific mobilization techniques for the stiff/fibrotic zygapophyseal/costotransverse joints of the thorax. The restricted motion will be identified and the relevant findings on functional movement testing and arthrokinematic testing outlined.

Bilateral Restriction of Flexion

The upper thorax is rarely fixed in a lordotic position, however, a bilateral restriction of flexion is not uncommon at T2-3 or throughout the vertebrosternal region generally (Fig. 4.3). Forward bending of the head/trunk reveals a limitation of the superior excursion of the transverse processes bilaterally and this can be confirmed on passive physiological mobility testing. The superior arthrokinematic glide at the zygapophyseal joint is restricted bilaterally.

Vertebromanubrial region

Longitudinal traction of the upper thorax will produce a superior glide of the zygapophyseal joint bilaterally. This technique is done with the patient supine lying. With the lateral aspect of the MCP of the index finger, the interspinous space is palpated at the level to be tractioned. With an open pinch grip of the other hand, the lower cervical spine is palpated as close to the superior vertebra of the level to be tractioned as possible (Fig. 6.1). Localization is achieved by flexing/extending the dysfunctional segment until the neutral position is ascertained. Grades 3 to 4 sustained longitudinal traction is applied by fixing the caudal vertebra and pulling the cranial vertebra superiorly.

Alternately, distraction can be done with the patient either sitting or standing with both hands behind the neck, fingers interlaced. The therapist winds both of their arms beneath the patient's axillae through the triangular space created by the flexed elbows. The fingers are interlaced and placed over the patient's hands (Fig. 6.2). The thorax is gently gripped by adducting the arms. The patient is instructed to look forward and the therapist ensures that the ligamentum nuchae is not on full stretch. From this position, a Grade 3 to 4 longitudinal traction technique is applied by rocking the patient backwards and forwards until a pendular type motion is produced. Gravity provides the distractive force. A high velocity, low amplitude thrust technique (Grade 5) can be applied at the apex of the descent when the patient's body weight is dropping.

To maintain the mobility gained, the patient is instructed to perform the following exercise. With the fingers interlaced behind the neck and the index fingers in the appropriate interspinous space, the patient is instructed to flex the head/neck. The fingers may assist the motion by applying a superior pressure to the inferior aspect of the spinous process of the superior vertebra. The amplitude of the exercise should be in the painfree range and should not aggravate any symptoms.

Vertebrosternal/vertebrochondral region

Longitudinal traction will produce a superior glide of the zygapophyseal joint bilaterally. This technique may be done with the patient either supine lying or sitting. The supine technique is performed as follows. The patient is sidelying, the head supported on a pillow and the arms crossed to the opposite shoulders. The therapist stands, facing the patient's head with their feet/legs in a stride position. With the tubercle of the scaphoid bone and the flexed PIP joint of the long finger, the transverse processes of the inferior vertebra are palpated. The other hand/arm lies across the patient's crossed arms to control the thorax (Fig. 6.3). Segmental localization is achieved by flexing the joint to the motion barrier with the hand/arm controlling the thorax. This localization is maintained as the patient is rolled supine only until contact is made between the table and the dorsal hand. From this position, further localization is achieved by compressing the thorax by adducting the dorsal arm, the hand of which is stabilizing the inferior vertebra of the segment to be mobilized. Longitudinal traction is applied through the thorax by shifting weight from the therapist's back leg/foot to the front leg/foot. The therapist's hand/arms focus the technique to the specific segment while the trunk/legs produce the mobilization force which is graded according to the needs of the joint. The technique can be graded from 3 to 5, the stiff joint will require a sustained grade 4 technique.

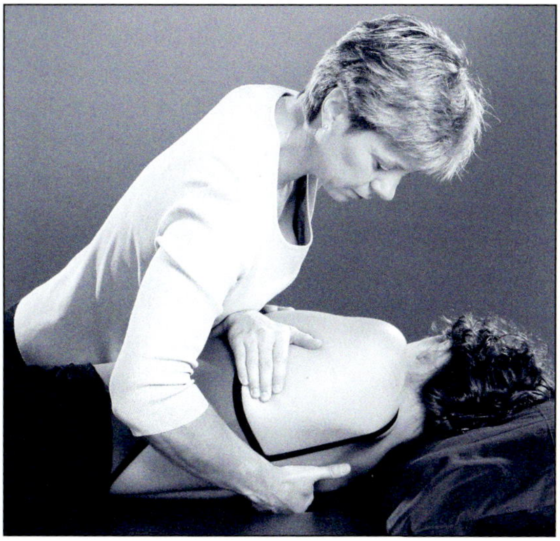

Figure 6.3. Bilateral flexion restriction – vertebrosternal and vertebrochondral region. Specific longitudinal traction – supine.

Distraction can also be applied with the patient sitting with the arms crossed to opposite shoulders. A small towel is placed against the spinous process of the caudal vertebra of the segment to be distracted. The towel is fixed against the therapist's sternum. With both arms wrapped around the patient's trunk, the patient's elbow which is closest to the chest is grasped (Fig. 6.4). The segment is

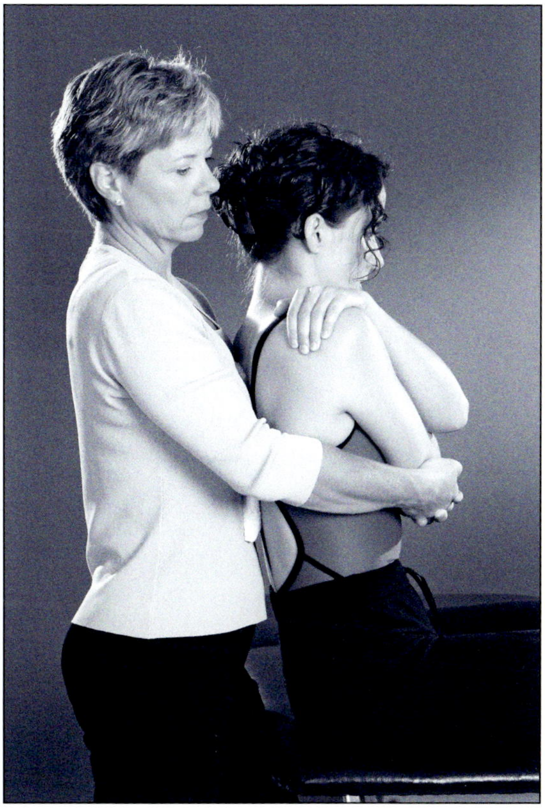

Figure 6.4. Bilateral flexion restriction – vertebrosternal and vertebrochondral region. General longitudinal traction – sitting.

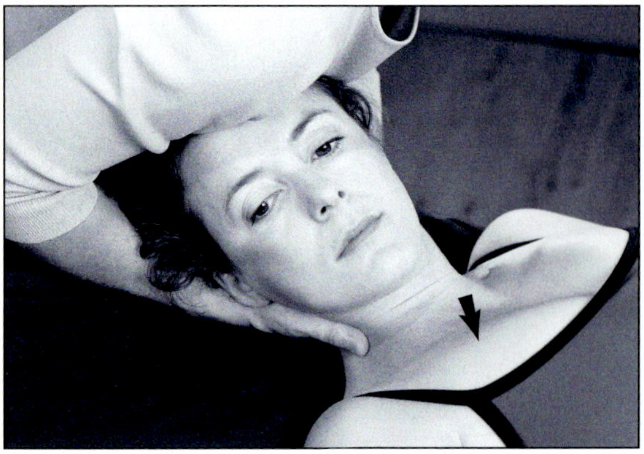

Figure 6.5. Unilateral flexion restriction – vertebromanubrial region. Right zygapophyseal joint T1-2.

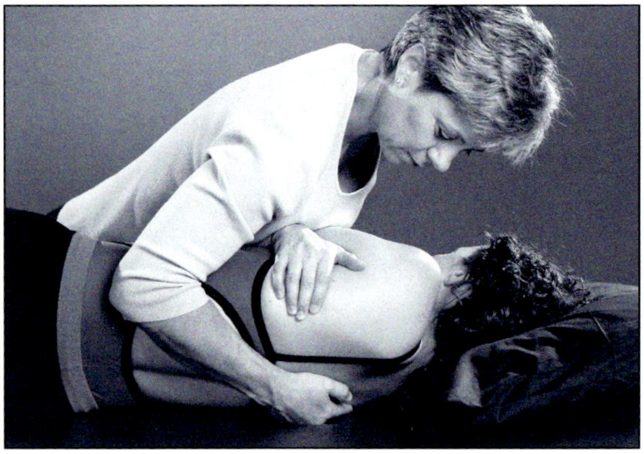

Figure 6.6. Unilateral flexion restriction – vertebrosternal and vertebrochondral region. Left zygapophyseal joint T5-6.

localized to neutral. From this position, distraction is applied by rocking the patient backwards and simultaneously lifting the thorax posterosuperiorly. The towel fixes the caudal vertebra and assists in localizing the distractive forces to the appropriate segment. The technique can be graded from 3 to 5.

Unilateral Restriction of Flexion

This is a common restriction to find in all regions of the thorax. Forward bending of the head/trunk reveals a limitation of the superior excursion of the transverse processes unilaterally and this can be confirmed on passive physiological mobility testing. The superior arthrokinematic glide at the zygapophyseal joint is restricted unilaterally.

Vertebromanubrial region – restricted flexion right T1-2

The patient is supine lying with the head supported on a pillow. With the lateral aspect of the index finger, the left transverse process of T1 is palpated. With the other hand, the midcervical spine is supported down to C7. The motion barrier is localized by passively flexing T1-2 and then gliding the left transverse process of T1 inferomedially on T2. C7-T1 is stabilized with the opposite hand by sideflexing the C7-T1 segment to the left and rotating it to the right. From this position, the right zygapophyseal joint of T1-2 is mobilized into flexion through an inferomedial and slightly posterior glide with the LEFT hand (Fig. 6.5). This will result in a superior and slightly anterior glide of the right facet at T1-2. The technique can be graded from 1 to 5, the stiff joint will require a sustained grade 4 technique.

Vertebrosternal/vertebrochondral region – restricted flexion left T5-6

The patient is right sidelying, the head supported on a pillow and the arms crossed to the opposite shoulders. The therapist stands, facing the patient's head with their feet/legs in a stride position. With the tubercle of the right scaphoid bone and the flexed PIP joint of the right long finger, the left transverse process of T6 and the right transverse process of T5 are palpated. The other hand/arm lies across the patient's crossed arms to control the thorax (Fig. 6.6). Segmental localization is achieved by flexing the joint to the motion barrier with the hand/arm controlling the thorax. This localization is maintained as the patient is rolled supine only until contact is made between the table and the dorsal hand. From this position, further localization is achieved by compressing the thorax by adducting the dorsal arm, the hand of which is stabilizing the inferior vertebra of the segment to be mobilized. From this position, a right sideflexion force is applied through the thorax to produce a superior glide of the left zygapophyseal joint. The technique can be graded from 1 to 5, the stiff joint will require a sustained grade 4 technique.

Thoracolumbar region – restricted flexion right T11-12

With the patient in left sidelying, hips and knees slightly flexed, the T10-11 interspinous space is palpated. The thoracolumbar spine is rotated by pulling/guiding the patient's lower arm forward until full rotation of T10-11 is achieved. The L1-2 interspinous space is palpated and the patient's uppermost hip and knee are flexed until full flexion of L1-2 occurs. The foot of the upper leg rests against the popliteal fossa of the lower leg. The T11-12 interspinous space is palpated and the right zygapophyseal joint is localized and mobilized into flexion and left sideflexion through either the thorax or the pelvic girdle (Fig. 6.7). The technique can be graded from 1 to 5, the stiff joint will require a sustained grade 4 technique.

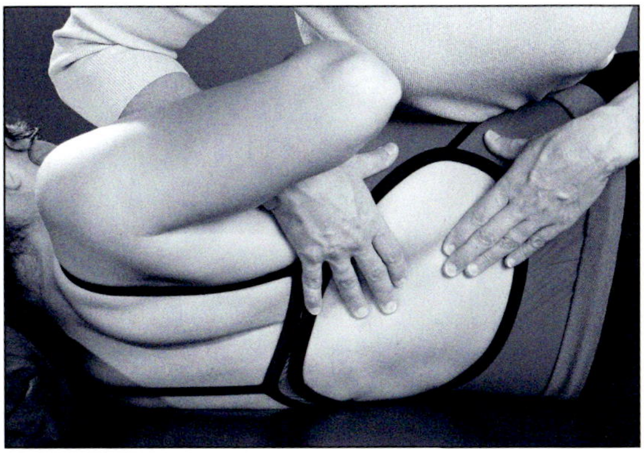

Figure 6.7 Unilateral flexion restriction – thoracolumbar region. Right zygapophyseal joint T11-12.

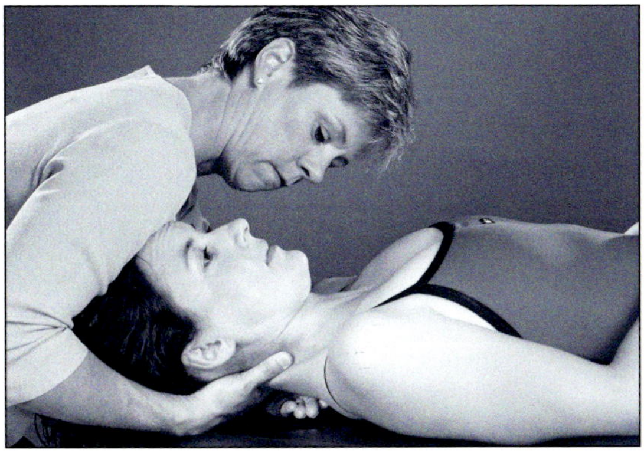

Figure 6.8. Bilateral extension restriction – vertebromanubrial region.

Bilateral Restriction of Extension

This restriction is commonly seen when the patient has a forward head posture and/or a collapsed, kyphotic thoracic posture. Bilateral elevation of the arms or extension of the midthorax will reveal a limitation of the inferior excursion of the transverse processes bilaterally. The inferior arthrokinematic glide at the zygapophyseal joint is restricted bilaterally.

Vertebromanubrial region

The patient is supine lying with the head supported on a pillow. With the lateral aspect of the index finger of one hand, the interspinous space is palpated at the level to be treated. The opposite hand supports the lower cervical spine as close to the segment as possible (Fig. 6.8). The motion barrier is localized and passively mobilized by dorsally gliding and slightly extending the superior vertebra. The technique can be graded from 1 to 4.

Unilateral Restriction of Extension

This is another common restriction to find in all regions of the thorax. Bilateral elevation of the arms or backward bending of the trunk reveals a limitation of the inferior excursion of the transverse process unilaterally and this can be confirmed on passive physiological mobility testing. The inferior arthrokinematic glide at the zygapophyseal joint is restricted unilaterally.

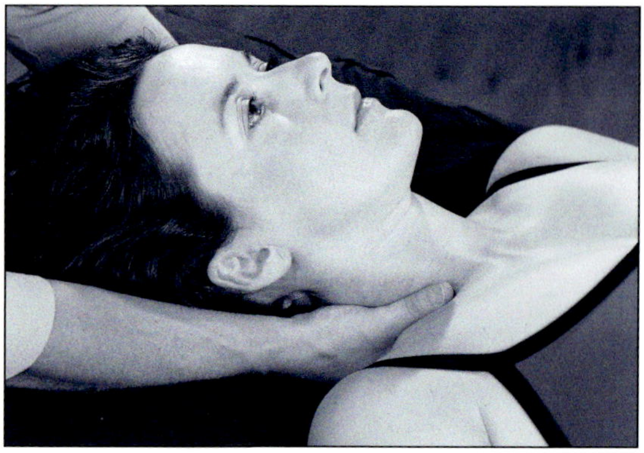

Figure 6.9. Unilateral extension restriction – vertebromanubrial region. Right zygapophyseal joint T1-2.

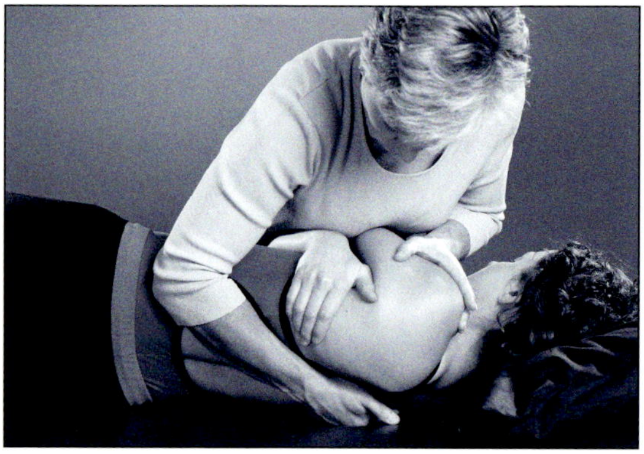

Figure 6.10. Unilateral extension restriction – vertebrosternal and vertebrochondral region. Left zygapophyseal joint at T5-6.

Vertebromanubrial region – restricted extension right T1-2

The patient is supine lying with the head supported on a pillow. With the lateral aspect of the index finger, the right transverse process of T1 is palpated. The midcervical spine is supported down to C7 with the other hand. The motion barrier is localized by passively extending T1-2 and then gliding the right transverse process of T1 posteroinferomedially on T2 (Fig. 6.9). C7-T1 is stabilized with the opposite hand by sideflexing the C7-T1 segment to the right and rotating it to the left. From this position, the right zygapophyseal joint of T1-2 is mobilized into extension through a posteroinferomedial glide with the RIGHT hand. The technique can be graded from 1 to 5, the stiff joint will require a sustained grade 4 technique.

Vertebrosternal/vertebrochondral region – restricted extension left T5-6

The patient is right sidelying, the head supported on a pillow and the arms crossed to the opposite shoulders. The therapist stands, facing the patient's head with their feet/legs in a stride position. With the tubercle of the right scaphoid bone and the flexed PIP joint of the right long finger, the left transverse process of T6 and the right transverse process of T5 are palpated. The other hand/arm lies across the patient's crossed arms to control the thorax (Fig. 6.10). Segmental localization is achieved by extending the joint to the motion barrier with the hand/arm controlling the thorax. This localization is maintained as the patient is rolled supine only until contact is made between the table and the dorsal hand. From this position, further localization is achieved by compressing the thorax by adducting the dorsal arm, the hand of which is stabilizing the inferior vertebra of the segment to be mobilized. From this position, a left sideflexion force (coupled with a slight dorsal glide) is applied through the thorax to produce an inferior glide of the left zygapophyseal joint. The technique can be graded from 1 to 5, the stiff joint will require a sustained grade 4 technique.

Thoracolumbar region – restricted extension right T11-12

With the patient left sidelying, hips and knees slightly flexed, the T10-11 interspinous space is palpated. The thoracolumbar spine is rotated by gently pulling/guiding the patient's lower arm forward until full rotation of T10-11 is achieved. The L1-2 interspinous space is palpated and the patient's uppermost hip and knee are flexed until full flexion of L1-2 occurs. The foot of the upper leg rests against the popliteal fossa of the lower leg. The T11-12 interspinous space is palpated and the right zygapophyseal joint is localized and mobilized into extension and right sideflexion through either the thorax or the pelvic girdle (Fig. 6.11). The technique can be graded from 1 to 5, the stiff joint will require a sustained grade 4 technique.

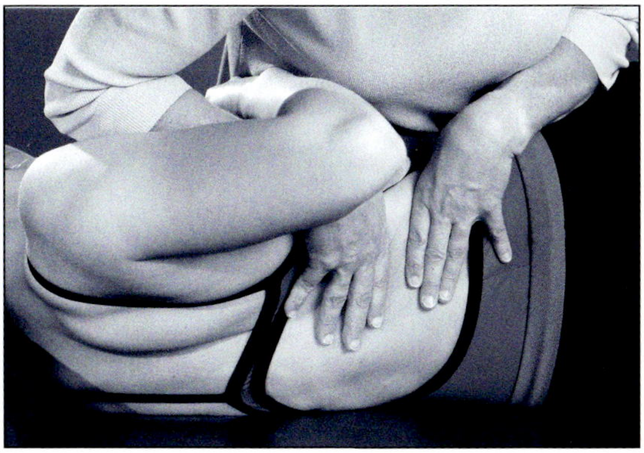

Figure 6.11. Unilateral extension restriction – thoracolumbar region. Right zygapophyseal joint T11-12.

Unilateral Restriction of Rotation – Rib

Vertebromanubrial region – restricted anterior rotation right 1st rib

This dysfunction will restrict extension of the head/neck. Rotation and lateral bending of the head/neck will be limited to the side of the restricted rib (this motion requires a superior glide of the rib at the costotransverse joint). Full expiration will also reveal asymmetry of rib motion. The superior glide of the first rib at the costotransverse joint is restricted.

The patient is supine lying with the head supported on a pillow. The superior aspect of the right transverse process of T1 is palpated with the right thumb. The index and middle fingers of the right hand palpate the inferior aspect of the right first rib. The midcervical spine is supported with the other hand. The motion barrier is localized and mobilized by applying a posteroinferior glide to the transverse process of T1 (Fig. 6.12) thus producing a relative superior glide of the first rib at the costotransverse joint. The middle and index fingers of the right hand fix the inferior aspect of the first rib. The technique can be graded from 1 to 4, the stiff joint will require a sustained grade 4 technique.

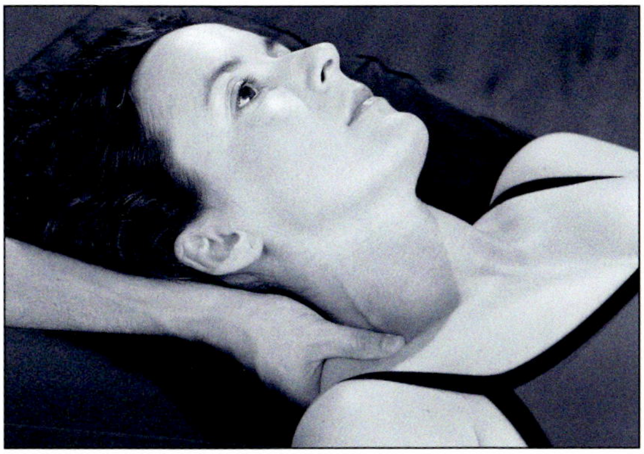

Figure 6.12. Unilateral anterior rotation restriction of the right first rib.

Vertebromanubrial region – restricted posterior rotation right 1st rib

This dysfunction will restrict flexion of the head/neck. Rotation and lateral bending of the head/neck to the opposite side of the restricted rib and full inspiration will also be limited. The inferior glide of the first rib at the costotransverse joint will be restricted.

The patient is supine lying with the head supported on a pillow. The superior aspect of the right first rib is palpated with the lateral aspect of the MCP of the index finger of the right hand. The midcervical and upper thoracic spine is supported with the other hand. The spine is stabilized by localized sideflexion of C7, T1 and T2 to the right and rotation to the left. The motion barrier of the first costotransverse joint is localized and mobilized by applying an inferior glide (Fig. 6.13) to the tubercle of the rib allowing the conjunct posterior

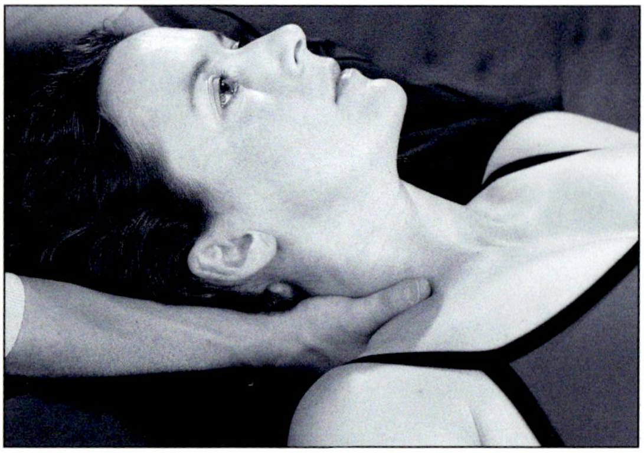

Figure 6.13. Unilateral posterior rotation restriction of the right first rib.

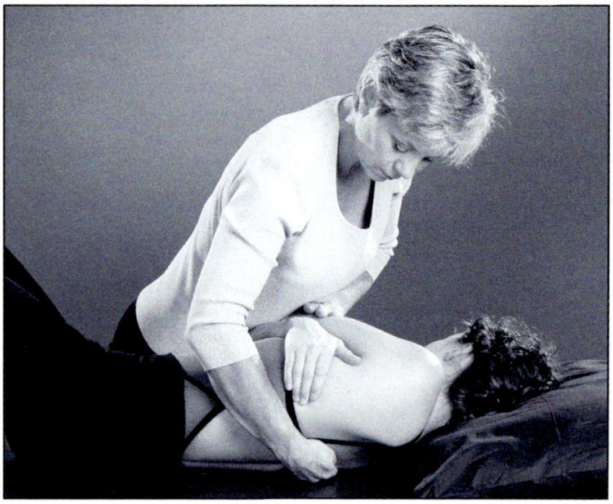

Figure 6.14. Unilateral rotation restriction of the left fifth costotransverse joint – distraction technique.

roll to occur. The technique can be graded from 1 to 5, the stiff joint will require a sustained grade 4 technique.

Vertebrosternal/vertebrochondral regions – restriction rib rotation

This dysfunction is seen when the costotransverse joint is restricted. It is common to see both anterior and posterior rotation restricted when this joint is fibrotic and distraction of the joint is the most effective technique for mobilization.

To mobilize the left 5th costotransverse joint the following technique is used. The patient is right sidelying, the head supported on a pillow and the arms crossed to the opposite shoulders. The therapist stands, facing the patient's head with their feet/legs in a stride position. With the proximal phalanx of the right thumb, the left 5th rib is palpated just lateral to the transverse process of T5. The other hand/arm lies across the patient's crossed arms to control the thorax (Fig. 6.14). Segmental localization is achieved by flexing the joint to the motion barrier with the hand/arm controlling the thorax. This localization is maintained as the patient is rolled supine only until contact is made between the table and the dorsal hand. From this position, further localization is achieved by compressing the thorax by adducting the dorsal arm, the hand of which is stabilizing the rib. From this position, further rotation of the localized thorax over the fixating thumb distracts the costotransverse joint. The technique can be graded from 1 to 5, the stiff joint will require a sustained grade 4 technique.

EXCESSIVE ARTICULAR COMPRESSION – COMPRESSED JOINT

The compressed joint will present with the following objective findings.

1. **Postural analysis.**
   The impact of a compressed joint on an individual's posture depends on whether the compression is confined to a single segment or spans multiple segments. A segmental joint compression may not reveal itself through postural analysis. Alternately, it may stand out as a segmental rotation in the midst of an otherwise normal curve. Multisegmental compression tends to alter the primary thoracic curve and can be exaggerated (kyphosis), reduced (lordosis) or twisted (rotoscoliosis).

2. **Functional movement tests and active mobility tests of osteokinematic function.**
   The pattern of motion on repeated testing can be variable depending on the irritability of the segment. A joint which is intermittently compressed may present with a variable pattern, changing from moment to moment and test to test. A joint which is under sustained compression (never lets go) will demonstrate a consistent pattern of motion on repeated testing.

3. **Articular function – form closure.**
   Once again, the pattern of restriction on segmental passive mobility testing can be variable with joints which are being compressed by the neuromyofascial system. While under compression, increased stiffness is palpable within the neutral zone and while the stiff joint has a solid end feel which does not vary with the speed of the test, the compressed joint is somewhat softer and the amplitude of motion can vary with the speed of the test. When the glide is applied rapidly, the amplitude of motion may be less than if the glide is applied slowly. This reflects the neuromyofascial cause of the articular compression. The passive tests for arthrokinetic function (passive stability) are often, but not always, normal.

4. **Neuromyofascial function – force closure and motor control.**
   The prone arm lift reveals poor thoracic position control.

5. **Neural conduction and mobility.**
   Conduction is normal and neural/dural mobility may or may not be restricted.

6. **Adjunctive tests.**
   X-rays are rarely helpful; they may reveal a rotoscoliotic or kypholordotic curve which is also evident on postural analysis.

Unilateral Restriction of Flexion/Right Sideflexion/Right Rotation

When the myofascia is overactive and compressing a left thoracic zygapophyseal joint the following release technique can be useful. The patient is sitting with the arms crossed to opposite shoulders. With the dorsal hand the intertransverse space is palpated. The ventral hand is placed on the contralateral shoulder. The motion barrier is localized by flexing and right sideflexing the thorax. From this position, the patient is instructed to hold still while the therapist applies gentle resistance to left rotation of the trunk (Fig. 6.15). The isometric contraction is held for up to 5 seconds following which the patient is instructed to completely relax. The new flexion/sideflexion barrier is localized and the mobilization repeated three times.

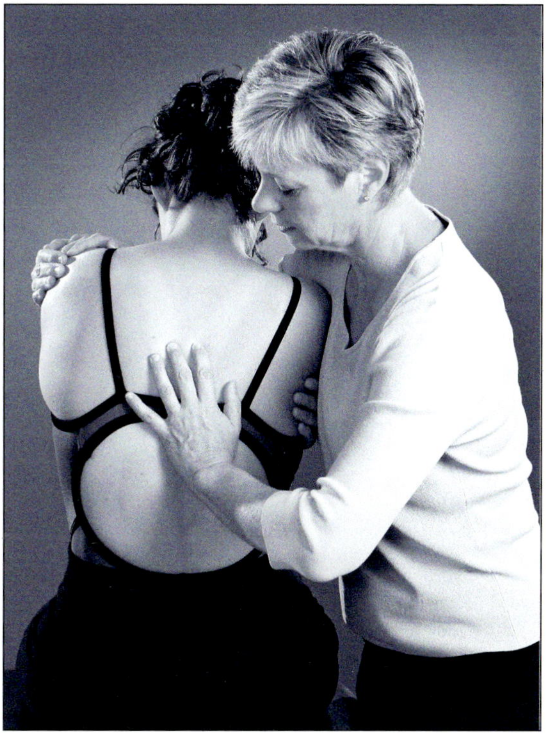

Figure 6.15. Unilateral restriction of flexion/right sideflexion/right rotation at T5-6 – release technique.

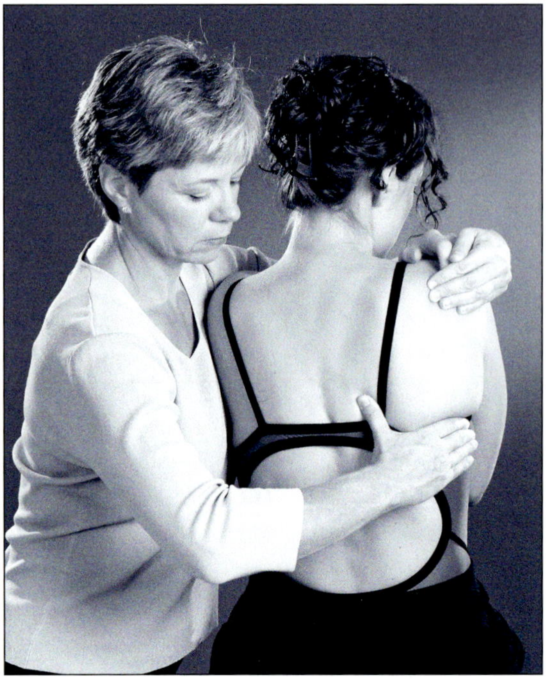

Figure 6.16 Unilateral restriction of posterior rotation of the right fifth rib – release technique.

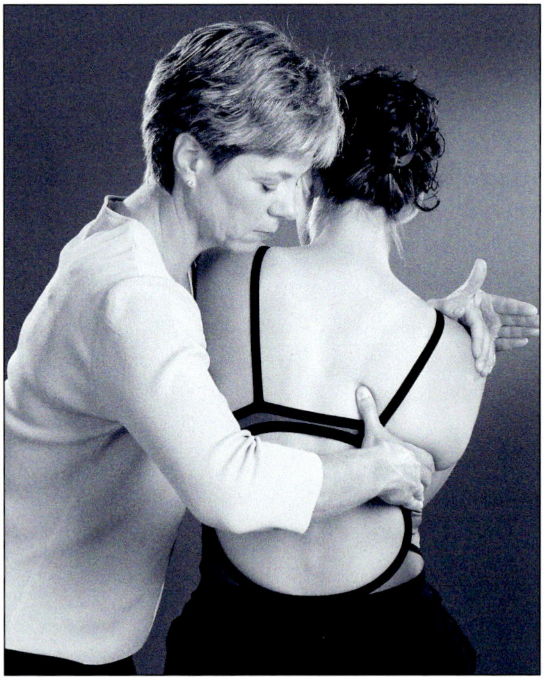

Figure 6.17 Unilateral restriction of anterior rotation of the right fifth rib – release technique.

Unilateral Restriction of Inspiration

When the myofascia is overactive and compressing the costotransverse joint the following release technique can be useful to restore posterior rotation of the right 6th rib. The patient is sitting with the arms crossed to opposite shoulders. With the dorsal hand the 6th rib is palpated. The ventral hand is placed on the patient's contralateral shoulder. The motion barrier is localized by left sideflexing and right rotating the thorax (Fig. 6.16). From this position, the patient is instructed to gently rotate the thorax against the therapist's resistance. The isometric contraction is held for up to 5 seconds following which the patient is instructed to completely relax. The new motion barrier is localized and the mobilization repeated three times.

Unilateral Restriction of Expiration

When the myofascia is overactive and compressing the costotransverse joint the following release technique can be useful to restore anterior rotation of the right 6th rib. The patient is sitting with the arms crossed to opposite shoulders. With the dorsal hand the 6th rib is palpated. The ventral hand is placed on the patient's contralateral shoulder. The motion barrier is localized by right sideflexing and left rotating the thorax (Fig. 6.17). From this position, the patient is instructed to gently rotate the thorax against the therapist's resistance. The isometric contraction is held for up to 5 seconds following which the patient is instructed to completely relax. The new motion barrier is localized and the mobilization repeated three times.

EXCESSIVE COMPRESSION WITH AN UNDERLYING INSTABILITY

A fixated joint is one which is unstable and is held compressed in an abnormal position by overactivation of muscles. The mode of onset is always traumatic. The location of the pain may be on the ipsilateral or contralateral side of the fixated joint and may radiate around or through to the anterior aspect of the chest. Breathing is commonly affected when the rib is fixated.

The fixated joint will present with the following objective findings.

1. **Postural analysis.**
   A "kink' or sudden deviation in the spinal or costal curve at the level of the fixation is easily noted.

2. **Functional movement tests and active mobility tests for osteokinematic function.**
   A consistent pattern of asymmetric motion is noted on repeated testing. Most movements of the thorax are effected in neither a zygapophyseal nor a costotransverse joint pattern.

3. **Articular function – form closure.**
   No motion is palpable. It is difficult to even find the plane of the joint for testing. Prior to manipulating the joint, the passive tests for arthrokinetic function (passive stability) are normal. After the joint has been decompressed (manipulative technique) the passive tests for arthrokinetic function reveal the underlying instability (neutral zone of motion is asymmetric and excessive compared to levels above and below).

4. **Neuromyofascial function – force closure and motor control.**
   The Prone Arm Lift test reveals poor thoracic position control. Manual compression of the thorax increases pain and increases the effort required to lift the arm.

5. **Neural conduction and mobility.**
   Conduction is normal and neural/dural mobility is often restricted.

6. **Adjunctive tests.**
   X-rays reveal a rotoscoliotic curve which is also evident on postural analysis.

The next section will describe/illustrate specific manipulation techniques for treating fixations of the costotransverse/costovertebral joint and the lateral shift lesion of the thoracic ring.

Fixation of the costotransverse/costovertebral joint

Vertebromanubrial region – superior fixation right 1st rib

The patient is supine lying with the head supported on a pillow. The superior aspect of the right first rib is palpated with the lateral aspect of the MCP of the index finger of the right hand. The midcervical and upper thoracic spine is supported with the other hand. The spine is stabilized by localized sideflexion of C7, T1 and T2 to the right and rotation to the left. The motion barrier of the first costotransverse joint is localized by applying an inferior glide to the tubercle of the rib. From this position a high velocity, low amplitude thrust is applied to the first rib in an inferior direction (Fig. 6.13).

Vertebrosternal/vertebrochondral region – fixation right 5th rib

The patient is right sidelying, the head supported on a pillow and the arms crossed to the opposite shoulders. The therapist stands, facing the patient's head with their feet/legs in a stride position. With the proximal phalanx of the right thumb, the left 5th rib is palpated just lateral to the transverse process of T5. The other hand/arm lies across the patient's crossed arms to control the thorax. Segmental localization is achieved by flexing the joint to the motion barrier with the hand/arm controlling the thorax. Distraction of the costotransverse joint is achieved by rolling the patient over the dorsal hand only until contact is made between the table and the dorsal hand. Further axial rotation of the thorax against the fixed rib will distract the costotransverse joint. A very low amplitude, high velocity thrust applied through the thorax in axial rotation will reduce the fixation (Fig. 6.14).

Thoracolumbar region – fixation right 12th costovertebral joint

Fixation of the eleventh or twelfth ribs at the costovertebral joint is not common given the flexibility of this region. A sudden contraction of the fully stretched quadratus lumborum muscle (hyperextension from the fully flexed position) can result in an inferior fixation of the twelfth rib. Excessive rotation of the trunk while fully flexed can also fixate these joints. When acute, the patient presents with a lateral shift of the trunk localized to the thoracolumbar junction. All active movements are blocked at the thoracolumbar junction. Any attempt to correct the lateral shift meets with resistance and an increase in the patient's pain.

With the patient in left sidelying, hips and knees slightly flexed, the T12-L1 interspinous space is palpated. The thoracolumbar spine is rotated by gently pulling/guiding the patient's lower arm forward until full rotation of T12-L1 is achieved. The L1-2 interspinous space is palpated and the patient's uppermost hip and knee are flexed until full flexion of L1-2 occurs. The foot of the upper leg rests against the popliteal fossa of the lower leg. The right side of the spinous process of T12 is palpated with the therapist's cranial hand. The right twelfth rib is palpated and fixed with the thumb and index finger of the therapist's left hand. The right costovertebral joint between the twelfth rib and T12 is distracted with a high velocity, low amplitude thrust technique by axially rotating the spinous process of T12 away from the fixed rib (Fig. 6.18).

Fixation of the 'Ring'

This fixation involves the entire 'ring' which includes two adjacent thoracic vertebrae, the intervertebral disc, the two ribs and their associated anterior and posterior joints and the sternum. This fixation occurs primarily in the vertebrosternal region and occasionally in the vertebrochondral region. It can occur when excessive rotation is applied to the unrestrained thorax or when rotation of the thorax is forced against a fixed rib cage (seat belt injury). At the limit of right rotation in the midthorax the superior vertebra has translated to the left, the left rib has translated posterolaterally and the right rib has translated anteromedially such that a functional U joint is produced (see biomechanics – Chapter 3). Further right rotation results in a right lateral tilt of the superior vertebra. Fixation

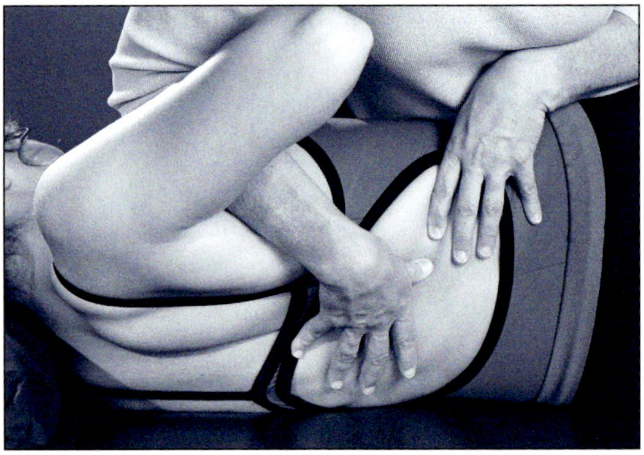

Figure 6.18. Thoracolumbar junction – unilateral fixation of the right twelfth rib at the costovertebral joint.

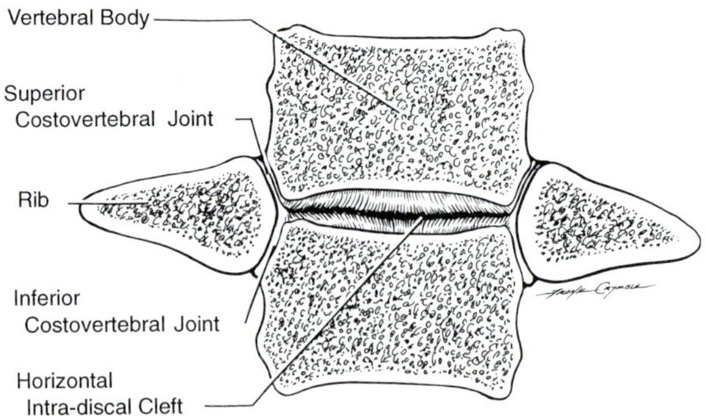

Figure 6.19. Anatomy of the lateral shift lesion. It is proposed that a horizontal cleft occurs through the posterior 1/3 of the intervertebral disc confluent with the superior costovertebral joints bilaterally allowing the superior vertebra to sublux laterally.

of the superior vertebra occurs when the left lateral translation exceeds the physiological motion barrier and the vertebra is unable to return to its neutral position. For the fixation to occur it is proposed that a horizontal cleft through the posterior 1/3 of the intervertebral disc must occur (Fig. 6.19).

Left lateral shift fixation of the 6th ring

1. **Postural analysis.**
   T5-T6 is right rotated, the right sixth rib is anteromedial posteriorly and the left sixth rib is posterolateral posteriorly.

2. **Functional movement tests.**
   All functional movements produce a 'kink' at T5-6, the most affected movement is rotation (Fig. 6.20).

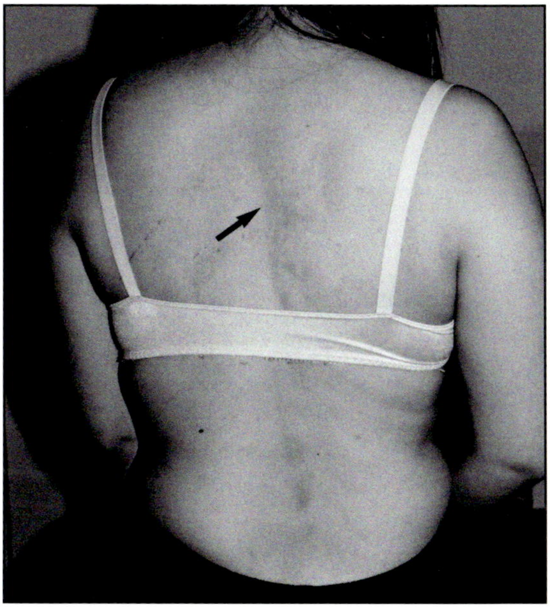

Figure 6.20. This patient sustained a lateral shift of T5 and the left and right sixth ribs in a motor vehicle accident one month prior. Note the complete block of right rotation at the fixated segment.

3. **Articular function – form closure.**
   There is a complete block to right lateral translation. Prior to manipulating the ring, the passive tests for arthrokinetic function (passive stability) are normal. After the segment has been decompressed (manipulative technique) the passive tests for arthrokinetic function for left lateral translation reveal the underlying instability (neutral zone of motion is asymmetric and excessive compared to levels above and below).

4. **Neuromyofascial function – force closure and motor control.**
   The Prone Arm Lift test reveals poor thoracic position control. Manual compression of the thorax increases pain and increases the effort required to lift the arm. After the segment has been decompressed, the left Prone Arm Lift will reveal a left lateral translation at T5-6. When manual compression is applied to the 6th ring, the effort required to lift the arm will be less and the lateral translation controlled.

5. **Neural conduction and mobility.**
   Conduction is normal and neural/dural mobility often restricted.

6. **Adjunctive tests.**
   X-rays reveal a rotoscoliotic curve which is also evident on postural analysis.

To release a left lateral fixation of the 6th ring, the following technique is used. The patient is in left sidelying, the head supported on a pillow and the arms crossed to the opposite shoulders. With the left hand, the right seventh rib is palpated posteriorly with the proximal phalanx of the thumb. T6 is fixed by compressing the right 7th rib towards the midline. Care must be taken to avoid fixation of the sixth ribs which must be free to glide relative to the transverse processes of T6. The other hand/arm lies across the patient's crossed arms to control the thorax. Segmental localization is achieved by flexing the joint until a neutral position of the zygapophyseal joints is achieved. This localization is maintained as the patient is rolled supine only until contact is made between the table and the dorsal hand. From this position, T5 and the left and right sixth ribs are translated laterally to the right through the thorax to the motion barrier. Strong longitudinal traction is applied through the thorax by shifting weight from the therapist's back leg/foot to the front leg/foot. This traction is maintained and a high velocity, low amplitude thrust is applied to the ring in a right lateral direction (Fig. 6.21). The goal of the technique is to distract and laterally translate T5 and the left and right sixth ribs relative to T6.

Once form closure has been restored to the joints of the thorax, attention should once again be directed to force closure analysis and motor control. The findings from these tests may be quite different than on the first evaluation so it is prudent to repeat these tests at this time. The next step in treatment is to ensure that force closure and motor control are restored. In the meantime, the thorax can be taped to prevent excessive translation during activities of daily living. Alternately, The Com-Pressor™ (Fig. 6.22) (www.optp.com) – a belt originally designed (D G Lee 2002) to assist in stabilization of the pelvic girdle can be used to apply a compressive force to the system. The body

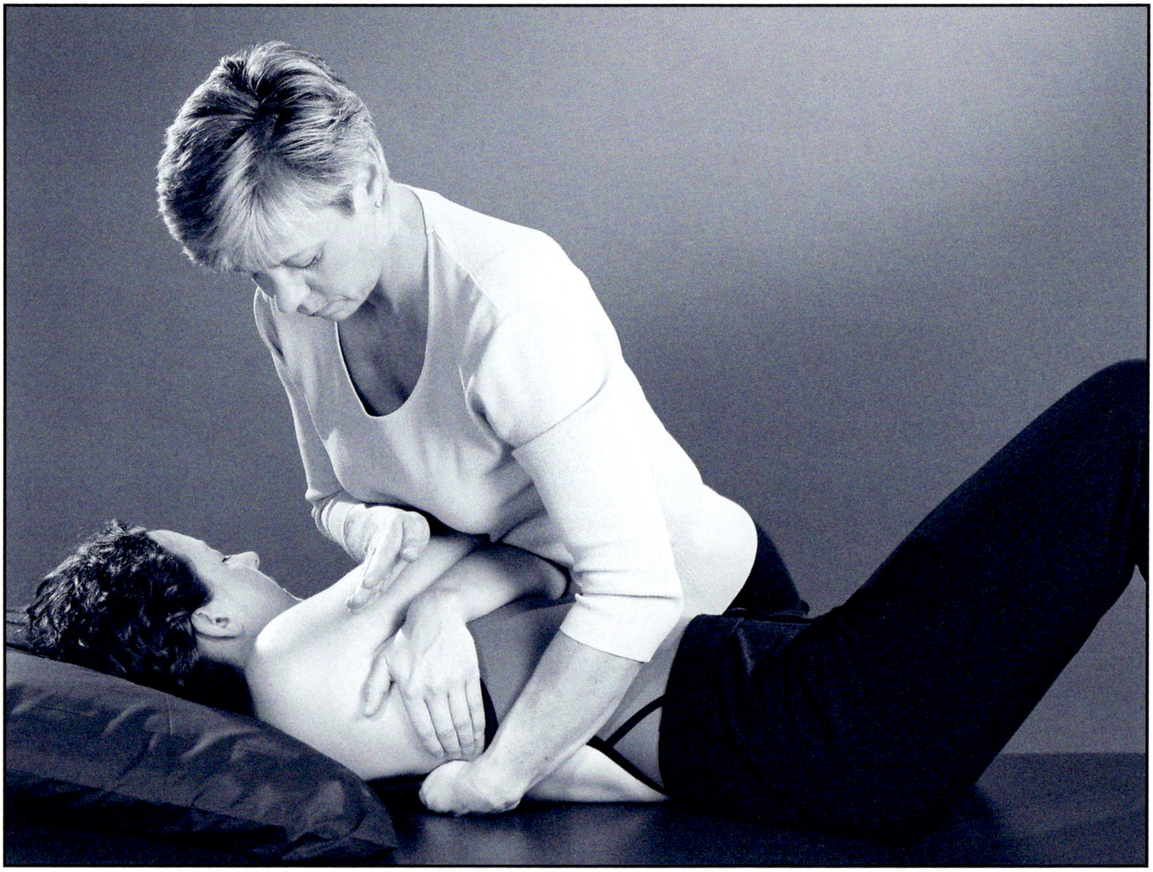

Figure 6.21. Manipulation technique for a left lateral shift of the sixth ring. Strong distraction must be maintained throughout the technique.

belt is applied around the thorax at the level of the unstable segment. The compression straps are applied to the body belt according to the findings of the Prone Arm Lift. If the effort required to lift the elevated arm is reduced when compression is applied posteriorly (approximating the ribs to the vertebra), then the straps are applied posteriorly to duplicate this compression force. If the anterior costochondral joints are unstable and anterior compression of the thorax during the Prone Arm Lift reduces the required effort to lift the elevated arm, then the straps are applied anteriorly to duplicate this compression force. The Com-Pressor™ should only be used to augment an exercise program (Chapter 7) for motor control.

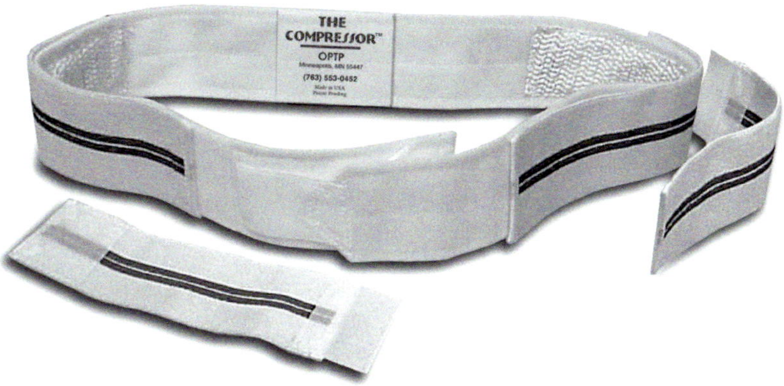

Figure 6.22. The Com-Pressor.

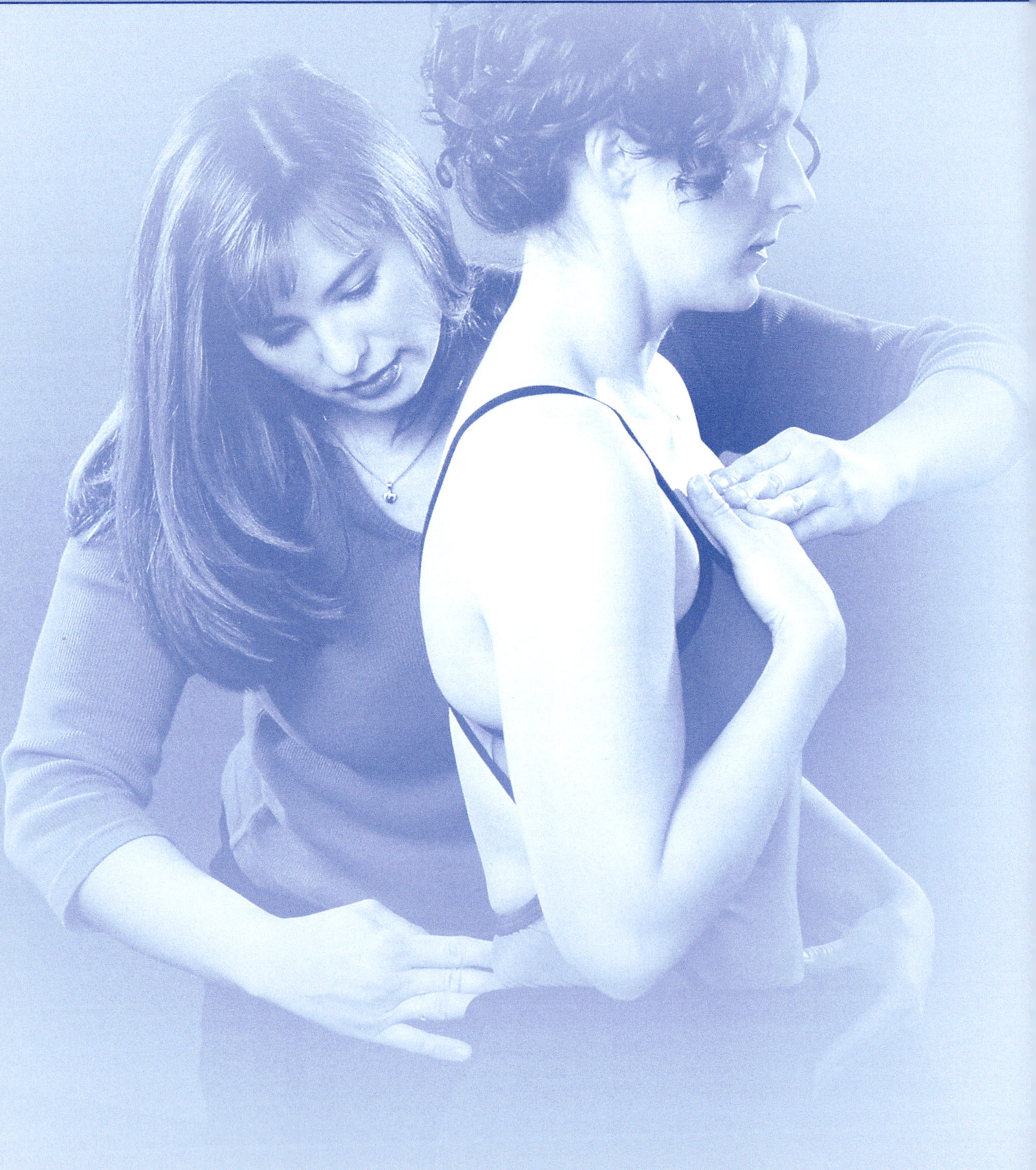

7

RESTORING FORCE CLOSURE/ MOTOR CONTROL OF THE THORAX

Written by Linda-Joy Lee

With respect to the thorax, it is the coordinated action between the local and global muscle systems that ensures stability without rigidity of posture and without episodes of collapse. This is the goal: "Mobility on Stability". The exercises presented in this chapter focus on balancing tension and compression forces and involve an extensive use of imagery. In this manner, individual muscles are recruited and appropriately timed for the coordinated execution and control of functional movement.

The reader is referred to the CD-ROM which accompanies this text to view short video clips of some of these exercises.

Chapter author's note: The concepts and exercises presented in this chapter are based on principles and ideas published in the work of many innovative researchers and clinicians such as Richardson, Jull, Hodges & Hides (1994 – 2000), Comerford & Mottram (2001), O'Sullivan (1997), Sahrmann (2001), and Janda (1978). My ideas have also been influenced by numerous discussions with skilled clinicians that I have been privileged to work with and learn from in my career. I am grateful for the many talented instructors of the Canadian Orthopaedic Division; in this system my manual therapy skills and clinical reasoning framework were cultivated. Ultimately, it is my patients who have continually pushed the development of these ideas, as their unique presentations require continual refinement and problem solving to help them reach their goals. I would like to thank Dr. Paul Hodges for his help with some of the figures in this chapter, and more importantly for his encouragement to pursue creative thinking while critically examining the evidence and asking relevant questions. Finally, I would like to thank Diane Lee for her support and the opportunity to present these ideas; her inexhaustible energy, enthusiasm, and commitment to fostering the growth of all those around her is a continual inspiration.

INTRODUCTION

Recent research has increased our understanding of muscle and joint function and consequently changed the way exercises for back pain and dysfunction are prescribed (Bergmark 1989, Bullock-Saxton et al 1993, Danneels et al 2000, Hides et al 1994, 1996, Hodges et al 1996, 1997a,b, 2000, Jull & Richardson 2000, Moseley et al 2002, O'Sullivan at al 1997, Richardson et al 1999). New concepts of how joints are stabilized and how load is transferred through the body highlight the importance of proprioception, automatic muscle activity, and motor control for regaining optimal movement after injury. It is clear from this body of evidence that successful rehabilitation of back pain and dysfunction requires exercises that differ from those used for conditioning and training the healthy, non-painful, non-injured population.

Patients typically present themselves to the clinician for two reasons: pain, and/or loss of function. Several studies (Bullock-Saxton et al 1994, Dangaria & Naesh 1998, Hides & Richardson 1996, Hodges & Richardson 1996, Mattila et al 1986, Uhlig et al 1995) have shown that changes in muscle fiber type, muscle bulk, and recruitment patterns occur with pain and pathology. However, simply relieving pain does not necessarily restore optimum function; these changes can remain even when pain subsides (Hides & Richardson 1996, Bullock-Saxton et al 1994). Changes in the proprioceptive and motor control systems alter movement patterns and strategies of load transfer. The result is less efficient movement, sub-optimal function, a higher risk for recurrence of pain and injury (Hides et al 2001), and altered joint forces (due to altered axes of joint rotation) that may lead to earlier degenerative changes and pain.

When planning injury rehabilitation, exercises should be prescribed as part of an integrated treatment plan, not as a stand alone treatment. If exercise is prescribed without first restoring form closure (Chapter 6) then the patient's pain and dysfunction often gets worse. This may then lead to the conclusion that certain exercises are "bad" or "unsuccessful" in treating back pain, when really it may be a problem of inappropriately timed exercise intervention.

Similarly, the type of exercise intervention is of utmost importance. A common theme arising from the evidence cited above is one of correcting deficits in motor control rather than focusing on strength and power of individual muscles. Patients who go mindlessly through a routine of exercises will have limited success in retraining motor patterns and may get worse with exercise if poor patterns and control are reinforced, resulting in irritation of joint structures and symptom exacerbation. It should be considered that the problem may not simply be WHICH exercise was prescribed, but HOW the exercise was performed. Three people performing a push up can do so with three different movement strategies, with three different combinations of muscle recruitment and timing. Therefore, when planning exercise intervention clinicians must remember that "exercise A" does not guarantee the use of "muscle A". It is up to the clinician to observe, assess, and decide if "exercise A" is reaching the goal of training "muscle A" (with appropriate recruitment, timing, endurance, etc.) for each patient. The key to correcting dysfunctional patterns of muscle activation is teaching awareness of movement; this requires mindfulness on the part of both the therapist and the patient.

With respect to the thorax, it is the coordinated action between the local and global muscle systems that ensures stability without rigidity of posture and without episodes of collapse. This is the goal: "Mobility on Stability". The exercises presented in this chapter focus on balancing tension and compression forces and involve an extensive use of imagery. In this manner, individual muscles are recruited and appropriately timed for the coordinated execution and control of functional movement.

CONCEPTS OF LOAD TRANSFER

The reader is referred to Chapter 2: Principles of the Integrated Model of Function for review of the definition of thoracic impairment and the components that contribute to functional stability.

To function optimally is to be able to maintain various postures and move freely in and out of these postures, without pain, and without unduly stressing the joints and surrounding soft tissues. Living in gravity requires transferring loads through the entire body and responding to ground reaction forces. To move and function in our environment, we also need to transfer loads to other objects under the force of gravity, as in lifting, pushing, and pulling. Thus, optimal function occurs when there is efficient and effective transfer of loads.

How does the spine transfer loads? Panjabi et al (1992) noted that the human spine depends on more than the simple stacking of blocks for stability; the osseoligamentous spine (the passive system) was shown to buckle at a load of only 2 kg, far less than normal loads on the spine in standing. It is a well-coordinated active system that provides the capacity to transmit the large forces to which the spine is exposed (Panjabi 1992). The term "tensegrity" (tension + integrity) was coined by Buckminster Fuller to describe the transference of forces through a combination of tension and compression. He used tensegrity concepts to design, and ultimately construct, buildings such as the geodesic dome. These structures transmit loads through a combination of tension and compression, without bending moments or shear forces (Levin, 1997). Applying tensegrity to the human spine, the bony structures (vertebrae, ribs) act as compression struts that are suspended by tension wires which are comprised of muscles, ligaments and fascia. The beauty of this system is its adaptability; finely tuned motor control allows alteration in the tension of the myofascial tension "wires" or "slings" to fit the demands of an infinite number of load transfer requirements both through time and space.

As mentioned in Chapter 2, stability (or effective load transfer) is not only about *how much* a joint is moving, or *how resistant* structures are that restrict it, but about motion *control*, which allows load to be transferred smoothly. The exercises in this chapter aim to establish a balance between compression and tensegrity within the thorax and to retrain this balance through motion *control* such that loads are transferred through the thorax with adequate (not too much, nor too little) approximation of joint surfaces for the given load demands.

Optimal Load Transfer Through the Thorax

The thorax is a central area in the spine that transfers loads between the lower quadrant (lower extremities and lumbopelvis), and the upper quadrant (upper extremities and neck). This function is highlighted in athletic activities such as baseball pitching, where there is transmission of power from the lumbopelvic region and lower extremities, up through the thorax and into the upper extremity. The thorax needs to provide stablility as a base for the scapula and arm, and concurrently allow rotational mobility and transmission of power and torque from the lumbar spine, pelvis and legs. Occupational activities such as pushing, pulling, and lifting will place similar load transfer requirements on the thorax.

In order to regain function, the requirements for optimal load transfer through the thorax must be met. The variety of ways that the thorax transfers load can be categorized and assessed. Each individual must have:

- Optimal lumbopelvic function.
- The ability to attain neutral spinal alignment within the thorax and in relationship to the cervical and lumbosacral curves.
- The ability to consciously recruit and maintain a tonic, isolated contraction of the local stabilizers of the thorax to ensure segmental control (control of the neutral zone).
- The ability to maintain and control neutral spine alignment during increased loading from the upper or lower extremities.
- The ability to move in and out of neutral spine alignment (flex, extend, rotate, sidebend) without segmental or regional collapse.
- The ability to maintain all the above and perform functional, work specific, and sport specific movements.

Dysfunctional Load Transfer Through the Thorax

In the lumbopelvic region, it is common to see segmental inhibition of the local muscle system associated with a multisegmental overactivitation of the global system (Richardson et al 1999, Radebold et al 2000, Arendt-Nielsen et al 1996, Kaigle et al 2000). Clinically, this dysfunctional finding also occurs in the thorax. If the local stabilizers are not functional, low-load tasks such as walking, or sustained standing can cause joint irritation and/or pain due to poor control of the neutral zone. Over-activation of the global muscles produces increased compression and often results in pain and rigidity of movement, rather than 'mobility on stability'. The objective examination tests described in Chapter 4 will reveal specific levels and directions of hypermobility/instability in the thorax; these findings will direct where and how to cue the correction of segmental control during exercise. Multisegmentally, postural changes such as excessive kyphosis, lordosis, or rotoscoliosis are common and usually result from dysfunctional patterns in the global muscle system (see Figures 4.2, 4.3, 4.4). These common non-optimal postures are addressed by restoring and teaching an awareness of the neutral spine position and integrating the new posture into functional patterns. This chapter will present an exercise program aimed at restoring a neutral thoracic spine position followed by restoring the function of the segmental local muscle system. Next, the progressions for integration of the dysfunctional segment back into the thorax such that segmental control is ensured during movement will be described. Finally, exercises which focus on control of the thorax in relation to the lumbar spine, pelvis, legs, and upper extremities will be presented.

DEVELOPING THE EXERCISE PROGRAM

Before specific exercises can be described, it is important to discuss some key considerations for developing the program. The therapist should:

- Educate the patient as to the importance of a new approach to "exercise"; discuss what happens to the brain's programming of muscle coordination with pain and injury and the importance of practice, mindful movement, and incorporation into daily activities. It is helpful to remind patients that this is not really exercise but rather "changing the way you live in your body".
- Remind the patient that "Practice makes Permanent, not Perfect" to reinforce the importance of quality of movement, rather than quantity of exercise.
- Ensure that the exercise program is specific to the patient's needs and not generic. This requires that faulty movement patterns are identified. The therapist should have determined:
  - the levels of poor control
  - the direction(s) of poor control
  - the levels or regions of restricted mobility
  - the overactive/dominant global muscles or slings of muscles
  - the inactive/under-recruited muscles (local stabilizers) or slings of muscles (global muscles)
  - any specific muscle length/strength imbalances
- Design and modify the exercise program based on tissue health, tissue irritability and stage of healing. Speed of progression will depend on a number of factors including the capacity of the patient for learning new tasks.

Strength, endurance and power of the global trunk muscles are important components of muscle function that should be assessed and treated when identified as deficits. However, it is not the intent of this chapter to present exercises or protocols for these components as several sources exist on these topics (McArdle et al 1991, McGill 2002, Farrell et al 1994). Instead, the focus of the exercises presented is the restoration of motor control whereby under-recruited muscles are reactivated through a mind-body awareness and imagery. This connection and activation of under-recruited local and global muscles is essential prior to prescribing exercises for strength, as unless the brain is using the muscle, exercises given designed to strengthen that muscle will only serve to strengthen alternate muscles being substituted for the action (e.g. hip extension exercises for gluteus maximus can be performed using the hamstrings). Thus, the focus of the exercises here is control of movement, with optimum technique, and with an awareness of the segments and areas of poor control that need to be corrected. Once the brain has 'found' the muscle, protocols for endurance, strength and power can be used if needed for patient specific goals.

Altered muscle length has implications for strength (due to length-tension relationships) and for restriction of mobility. Assessment of the underlying cause of altered muscle length is crucial for correcting the dysfunction in the muscle. It is often not simply a matter of stretching a tight muscle. The exercises presented here are to be used in conjunction with techniques that restore functional length in muscles, and optimum performance of these exercises will be enhanced by such techniques.

THE EXERCISE PROGRAM

Introduction to Stabilization Exercises for the Lumbopelvic Region

A properly functioning lumbopelvic region serves as the base upon which the thorax moves and transfers load. When assessing the patient with thoracic dysfunction, it is important to include a screening examination of the lumbopelvic region, including tests such as the Active Straight Leg Raise (ASLR) (Mens et al 1997, 1999, Lee 1999) to determine if load transfer is effective and to observe the motor control strategies used by the patient. Poor lumbopelvic stabilization strategies will limit the patient's ability to attain and control optimal spinal postures (and thus optimal thoracic positions), as well as limit progression of the thoracic stabilization program to exercises that require thoracopelvic dissociation and control of neutral spine.

During the ASLR, some obvious signs that the local stabilizers of the lumbopelvic region need to be addressed include abdominal bracing and rigidity, bulging of the lower abdomen, breath holding, asymmetry of control between right and left legs, obvious difficulty in lifting one leg, and significant rotation/deviation of the pelvis to one side (Lee 1999, Richardson et al 1999).

The four muscles of interest are the diaphragm, transversus abdominis (TA), deep fibres of multifidus (dMF), and the pelvic floor (PF) (Figure 7.1, also see Chapter 2, Force Closure). Studies have shown that these deep local stabilizing muscles are anticipatory, non-direction specific, and maintain tonic contractions at low levels throughout activities. In dysfunction, the local muscles lose these characteristics and become delayed in their timing, direction specific, and phasic (Hodges & Richardson, 1996, Richardson et al 1999, Moseley et al 2002). To retrain the local system, patients are first taught to isolate and maintain a tonic contraction of the deep muscles, separate from the global muscles. This is artificial in the sense that in normal function, these local muscles work in conjunction with the global muscles. However, in dysfunction this coordinated action of the local and global systems is lost; in order to address the change in motor control strategy the local system must be trained separately. This protocol of isolation, training tonic holding ability, and then integration with global muscles and into functional activities is an effective means for retraining the coordinated function of the local system (O'Sullivan et al 1997, Hides et al 1996, 2001).

There are several techniques that can be used to facilitate isolation of the local muscle system, including education (anatomy of the muscles, their function, and the contrast between deep muscles and superficial muscles), decreasing

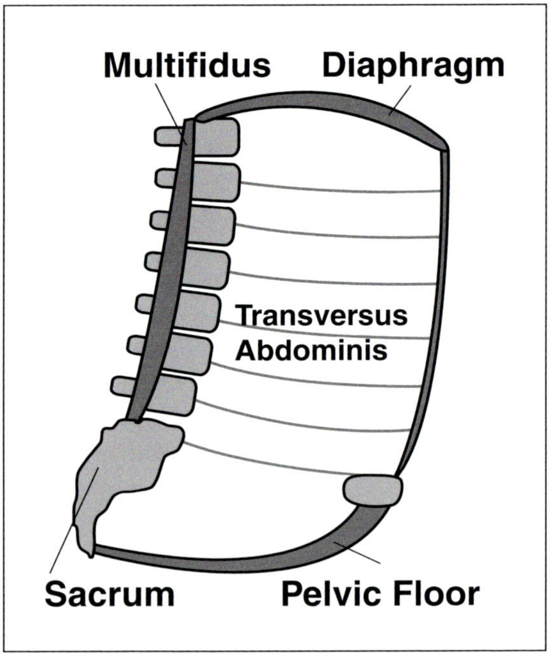

Figure 7.1 The local stabilizers of the lumbopelvic region. Optimal function of the thorax requires optimal function of the lumbopelvic region; proper recruitment of these muscles helps to facilitate isolation of the deep local stabilizing muscles for the thorax. Reproduced with permission from Lee 2001.

activity in the global muscle system, facilitation of neutral spine position, tactile feedback, and co-activation of other deep muscles (eg. PF contraction to facilitate TA). Along with these techniques, the use of images to help the patient re-establish the brain-body connection has been found to be very effective. In this section some images will be described for recruiting and isolating the transversus abdominis and the deep fibres of multifidus components of the lumbopelvic local stabilizing system. The pelvic floor component is discussed, and diaphragmatic function is addressed below in the breathing section of the stabilization program for the thorax. For those patients with thoracic dysfunction requiring a stabilization program, the images for recruitment of the lumbopelvic region can also be used to facilitate the deep muscles which stabilize the thorax. The two systems appear to function harmoniously.

The material here is a brief overview on the topic of lumbopelvic segmental stability; the reader is referred to Richardson, Jull, Hodges, and Hides' "Therapeutic Exercise for Spinal Segmental Stabilization in Low Back Pain" (1999), Diane Lee's "The Pelvic Girdle", 2nd edition (1999), and Diane Lee's "Imagery for Core Stabilization" video for more in depth background on assessing and training segmental stability for the lumbopelvic region.

Pelvic floor

Sapsford et al (2001) have shown that activation of the abdominal muscles should accompany contraction of the pelvic floor muscles and vice versa. Images and explanations that involve contraction of the anterior pelvic floor (pubococcygeus) are useful facilitation techniques for obtaining an isolated transversus abdominis (TA) contraction and are described below. Sapsford et al's research supports using a submaximal contraction of the pelvic floor in a position of neutral pelvic tilt to best facilitate contraction of TA. Training the tonic function of the pelvic floor muscles involves a slow, gentle, submaximal contraction, with a focus more anterior (vaginal or urethral) than posterior (rectal). However, it is important to recognize that if a successful isolated TA contraction occurs with verbal cueing of the pelvic floor, it can not be guaranteed that a proper contraction of the pelvic floor has occurred, especially in those patients with specific pelvic floor dysfunction (eg. stress incontinence, pain syndromes, trauma). Bump et al (1991) found that only 49% of female patients presenting in a gynecological and urodynamic laboratory could perform a correct pelvic floor contraction when given verbal or written instructions. Thus, if the therapist suspects either hypertonicity or poor recruitment of the pelvic floor musculature, a referral to a therapist specializing in pelvic floor dysfunction and manual assessment of the floor is recommended.

Transversus abdominis

Patient position: The initial position chosen to teach this exercise will depend on which position encourages relaxation of the global muscles while ideally providing some stretch on the abdominal wall for proprioceptive feedback. The best position for each patient will vary depending on their substitution strategies. For example, supine crook lying is most supportive and allows relaxation of global muscles such as the erector spinae; however, there is little stretch on the abdominal wall to provide feedback for the patient of where the "drawing in" action of TA should occur. The side lying position provides more stretch on the abdominal wall due to the pull of gravity on the abdomen. When a rolled towel is placed under the waist and a pillow inserted between the knees, the sidelying position can be a supportive position to allow global muscle relaxation. The 4-point kneeling position is a good starting place to help the patient understand the feeling of "drawing in" the lower abdomen. Depending on the substitution strategies observed, a more supported position may be the subsequent choice for further training of an isolated contraction of TA. Ideally, a neutral position for the lumbar spine should be attained (avoid a flexed, flat lumbar spine and posterior pelvic tilt) since the neutral spine position is known to facilitate the isolation of TA (Sapsford et al 2001), especially in patients exhibiting a dominance of the oblique muscles.

Therapist position: Palpate the abdomen 2.5 cm medial to and slightly inferior to the ASIS (anterior superior iliac spine) bilaterally (see Figure 7.2). The patient should be taught how to palpate here for a proper contraction. In sidelying, the therapist can also gently cup the lower abdomen with the palm to provide feedback of where the contraction should be initiated. Observe the abdominal wall and trunk for signs of proper isolation without global muscle activation.

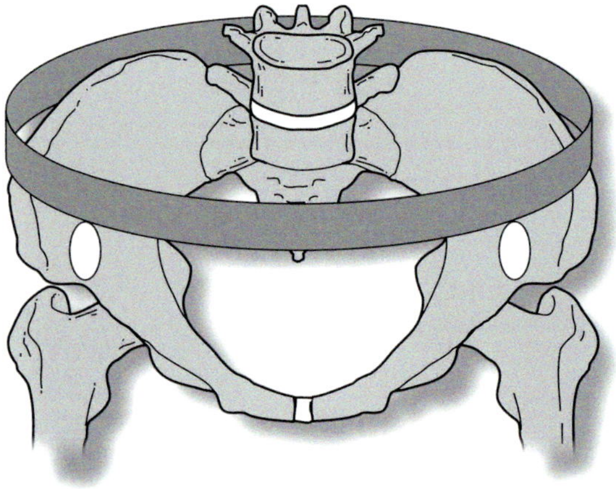

Figure 7.2 The oval circles just medial to the ASIS on each side indicate the points for palpating contraction of transversus abdominis. An isolated contraction will be felt as a slow, gentle flattening and tensioning under the fingers. Any bulge or rapid contraction is evidence of contraction of the internal oblique. The circle around the pelvis represents the corseting action produced by the co-contraction of transversus abdominis and the deep fibres of multifidus. Reproduced with permission from Lee 2001.

Therapist facilitation: Verbal cues

"Breathe in, breathe out, then don't breathe as you slowly, gently draw your lower abdomen away from my fingers (or hand)"

"Imagine that there is a slow tension coming up from the inner thighs into the front of your pelvic floor, then extend that tension up into my fingers in your lower abdomen"

"Imagine that you are slowly and gently drawing these two bones (ASIS's) together"

"Very lightly and slowly think of lifting up in your pelvic floor" (for women can imagine lifting the vagina, for men doing a small lift of the testes).

Therapist facilitation: Manual cues

Provide a sinking pressure into the abdomen as you give the verbal cues slowly and gently. Tactile pressure can also be given just above the pubic bone or with the hand cupping the abdomen; sink into the tissue slowly to encourage a slow, tonic contraction instead of a fast, phasic response. If there is excessive upper abdominal activity, the patient can continue to palpate at the ASIS points while the therapist provides gentle tactile pressure bilaterally into the upper medial thighs to take the focus away from the stomach and imagine the contraction starting lower.

Ideal response: A slow development of gentle tensioning under the fingers should be felt. It should be remembered that only a 15-20% contraction of this muscle is required. If the patient uses too much effort or performs a fast contraction, a bulge into the fingers will be felt, pushing the fingers away from the abdomen; this is the internal oblique (IO) muscle. There should be no pelvic or spinal movement, and little movement in the upper abdomen. Rectus abdominis and the obliques should remain relaxed. If the rib cage is depressed and drawn in, this is a sign of external oblique activation. Perform a small "wiggle" of the rib cage by pushing it gently laterally; if there is a lot of resistance to your pressure this means the rib cage is being braced by overactive global muscles and an isolated TA contraction has not been achieved. The rib cage should still move easily in response to the lateral pressure in the presence of an isolated TA contraction.

Progressions/Other considerations:

- When an isolated contraction has been achieved, ask the patient to maintain the contraction while breathing normally. The eventual goal is a 10 second hold, for 10 repetitions.
- The absence of spinal movement (eg. pelvic tilt) does not necessarily mean that TA has been isolated. A co-contraction of the internal and external obliques along with the erector spinae will result in no aberrant spinal motion, but will restrict rib cage movement and the ability to perform lateral costal expansion during breathing. It is important to use your hands and eyes to assess for signs of global muscle substitution during the contraction.
- Using your voice in a slow, gentle manner will facilitate a better pattern.
- Consider asking the patient to reduce the effort of the contraction and to reduce the speed to facilitate TA isolation.
- Once the patient is able to sustain a tonic contraction of TA for 10 seconds, the exercise can be progressed. Specific strategies for these progressions are described elsewhere (Lee 2001, Richardson et al 1999). The principles to consider when progressing these exercises are to ensure that there is a pre-contraction of the local system and then adding:
  - coordination with breathing
  - co-contraction with dMF and PF
  - adding the global muscles while maintaining a neutral spine position
  - moving out of neutral spine position with global muscle activity
  - integration into functional activities

Deep fibres of multifidus

Patient position: Prone or sidelying are good positions as they allow relaxation of the erector spinae and access for palpation of the multifidus muscle. However, positions such as supine can also be beneficial for some patients.

Therapist position: Palpate multifidus just lateral to the spinous processes of the lumbar spine bilaterally at the level of atrophy. To monitor the deep fibres, the muscle must be palpated close to the spine; in the lower lumbar segments the lateral muscle bulk consists of the more superficial fibres. Teach the patient how to find the dysfunctional segment and how to sink into the muscle with the fingers.

Therapist facilitation: Verbal cues

"Feel the muscle under my finger, think of a tension coming from inside your body to make this muscle bulge into my fingers"

Barbie doll: "Imagine that you are a Barbie doll and that someone has pulled your leg off and left it lying at your pelvis, but disconnected. Imagine an energy from inside your spine that will draw the leg into your body and reconnect it". Or, "Imagine there is a string connected from the spine to the hip (in the groin), if you pull on this string from the muscle in your back you can connect the leg back into your body"

Guy wire/Tent wire: "Imagine that there is tent wire or string that is connecting from the front of your pelvic floor, up and in through your body diagonally to my fingers in your spine. Breathe in, breathe out, now slowly connect a wire from this finger here (give pressure at upper inner thigh) to this finger here (give pressure into multifidus)". "You are creating a tension in the wire to suspend the spine".

Therapist facilitation: Manual cues: The timing of the tactile pressure from the therapist's hands creates the image and provides feedback as to how quickly the muscle should be contracted. The fingers should sink into the multifidus and provide a cranial pressure to encourage a "lifted" or "suspended" feeling. For the tent wire images, the start of the wire can be just medial to the ASIS's, superior to the pubic bone, or from the pelvic floor; the sequence of tactile feedback is from the anterior palpation point first, then up into the multifidus palpation point.

Ideal response: A slow development of firmness in the muscle will be felt as an indentation of the pads of the palpating fingers. A fast contraction is indicative of superficial multifidus and/or erector spinae activation; the fingers will be quickly pushed off the body. It is important to teach the patient how easy it is to push the fingers into the muscle when it is relaxed ("feels like a mushy banana") as compared to when it is contracted ("feel how it is firmer and harder to sink your fingers into the muscle"). There should be no pelvic or spinal motion observed, and no activity in the global abdominal muscles or in the hip musculature. A co-contraction of TA is acceptable and desired.

Progressions/Other considerations:

- The image that is used for training the muscle depends on which image gives the best isolated contraction of deep multifidus. The patient is then instructed how to feel the contraction and how to monitor for any substitutions.
- When an isolated contraction has been achieved, ask the patient to maintain the contraction while breathing normally. The eventual goal is a 10 second hold, for 10 repetitions.
- Using your voice in a slow, gentle manner will facilitate a better pattern.
- Progressions are explained in detail in other sources (Lee 2001, Richardson et al 1999); the principles are to pre-contract the local system and then add:
  - coordination with breathing
  - co-contraction with TA and PF
  - adding the global muscles while maintaining neutral spine position
  - moving out of neutral spine position with global muscle activity
  - integration into functional activities

Stabilization of the Thorax

Optimal function requires segmental control at each thoracic level; that is, control of the neutral zone of motion for each thoracic segment. For the lumbar spine, it is well established that the muscles best suited to this function are the deep local muscles (transversus abdominis, deep fibres of multifidus, diaphragm, pelvic floor). There are comparatively few studies on the function of the deep muscles of the thoracic spine. Based on the anatomy of the thoracic region, it is hypothesized that the deep segmental muscles (rotatores, multifidus) will have a similar function in the thoracic region. Donisch and Basmajian (1972) qualitatively analysed EMG data from the deep muscles bilaterally at the level of the T6 and L3 spinous processes in different postures and range of movement tests. They concluded that the deep muscles in both regions acted as stabilizers rather than prime movers. Morris et al (1962) recorded EMG activity from the deep muscles lateral to the spinous process of T10. Qualitative analysis revealed variable patterning during different activities; however, the inter-electrode distance was large (2 cm), making the measurements less specific. Clearly more research in this area is needed. Clinically it has been the author's experience that there is often atrophy and loss of activation of these deep segmental muscles at the dysfunctional levels in the thorax, and that restoring the tonic function of these muscles is essential for regaining segmental stability. Thus, the first goal of this stabilization program is to teach an isolated contraction of the deep, segmental muscles at the level(s) of hypermobility. In order to reach this goal, the impact of the global muscle system must first be considered since excessive activity of the global system inhibits the ability to recruit the local system.

Many authors have noted patterns of global muscle hyperactivity and dominance (Sahrmann 2001, Hall & Brody 1999, Comerford & Mottram 2001, Janda 1978). A consistent finding in patients with low back pain is that there are one or more global muscles that are overactive, hypertonic, and dominant (Radebold et al 2000, Arendt-Nielsen et al 1995, Kaigle et al 2000). In the thoracic spine, the dominant global muscles include the thoracic erector spinae, the scapular muscles (rhomboids, levator scapulae, trapezius), the latissimus dorsi, the external and internal obliques, and the rectus abdominis. There are several methods that can be used to reduce global muscle tone, including using surface EMG as biofeedback for downtraining, dry needling or IMS (Intramuscular Stimulation, Gunn 1999), trigger point release, etc. The use of diaphragmatic breathing and neutral spine position can be very effective in reducing global muscle activity and preparing the motor system to learn new stabilization strategies. Thus, techniques to establish more optimal breathing patterns and spinal alignment are described here prior to starting segmental isolation of the deep thoracic stabilizing muscles.

Breathing

Optimal diaphragmatic breathing involves both abdominal and lower ribcage expansion (Detroyer 1989). The most common component lost in patients with thoracic dysfunction is lateral costal expansion. When lateral/posterolateral expansion is absent, excessive excursion occurs in the abdomen (making it difficult to attain a functional transversus abdominis contraction) or in the upper chest (associated with excessive accessory respiratory muscle activity). Also commonly present is hypertonicity and bracing with the external and/or internal oblique and/or the erector spinae muscles; the presence of this muscle activity then continues to restrict lower rib cage movement. Changing the pattern of inspiration can be used to release hypertonicity of these global muscles.

Under normal respiratory demand, expiration should be a passive action resulting from the elastic recoil of the chest and abdomen. Any evidence of active expiration by use of the abdominal muscles should be noted as this pattern can also reinforce restriction of mobility in the thoracic joints.

Patient position: Supine, crook lying.

Therapist technique: Before placing your hands on the patient, first observe and assess the habitual breathing pattern over several inspiration/expiration cycles. Look for movement in the upper chest (apical breathing), the lateral lower rib cage (lateral costal expansion), and the abdomen (upper and lower abdomen). Note the area where most movement occurs. Next, place your hands on the lateral aspect of the lower rib cage to monitor movement. Check for amount of movement and symmetry between the left and right sides.

Ideal pattern: Most of the movement on inspiration should occur in the lower lateral rib cage with concurrent movement of the upper abdomen. Retraining lateral costal expansion is an important component of the exercise program; it helps maintain mobility gained from the manual treatment at hypomobile levels (see Chapter 6) while facilitating the use of the deep local muscle system instead of the global system.

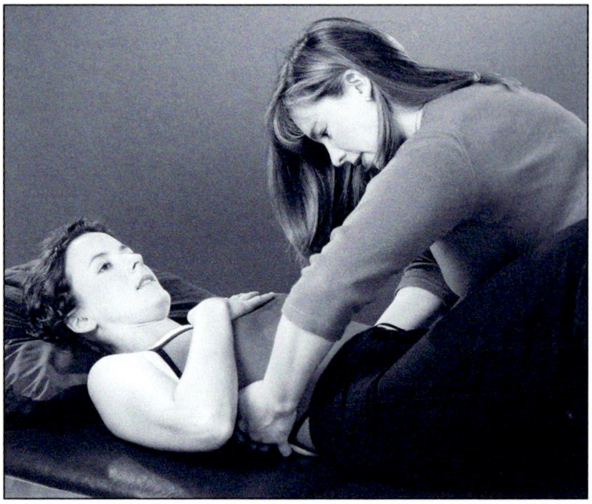

Figure 7.3 Correction Technique: Facilitation of Lateral Costal Expansion. The therapist uses gentle inward compression at the end of expiration to give feedback as to where the patient needs to direct their breath, and releases this pressure as the patient begins inspiration. In this example, the patient is using one hand to monitor for excessive apical chest movement. The hand can also be placed on the lower abdomen to monitor excessive movement there.

Correction technique: Keep your hands on the lateral aspect of the lower rib cage and give the patient an image to redirect their inspiration (see Figure 7.3).

Therapist facilitation: Verbal cues

"As you breathe in, imagine bringing the air into my hands"

"Imagine your ribs are like an umbrella, and when you breathe in the bottom of the umbrella is opening up"

"With each breath open your ribs into my hands"

For muscle activity on expiration:

"As you breathe out, let the air fall out of you and relax your stomach"

"Imagine I am slowly pulling the air out of you"

"Think of sighing the air out as you breathe out"

"Let your chest and sternum go heavy to the floor as you exhale"

Therapist facilitation: Manual cues: With your hands, apply a slow, gentle, inward pressure bilaterally at the end of expiration and release this pressure slightly after the start of the inspiration phase (rib springing). Allow your hands to follow the rib cage opening, then apply the gentle pressure again at the end of expiration. If the restriction of lateral costal expansion is asymmetrical, apply your pressure asymmetrically and have the patient mentally focus on the side of less excursion. To release excessive global tone on expiration, gently wiggle/rotate the rib cage a small amount to release the muscle holding as the patient expires.

Parameters & functional integration: The patient should perform focused breathing pattern retraining 2-3 times a day, using both normal and deeper breaths, for several minutes. The patient uses their own hands on the sides of the rib cage to provide self-feedback. Alternately, a theraband can be used around the lower rib cage for proprioceptive feedback; use the lowest resistance of band to allow flexibility and rib cage expansion. To encourage the transfer of the new breathing pattern into a more automatic strategy, have the patient "check-in" on their pattern at different points throughout the day, in different postures and during different activities (sitting, standing, walking, etc.).

Neutral spine

Sitting (see Figure 7.4, Video Clip 7.5)

Patient position: Sitting on a chair or a ball. If the patient has a restriction of hip flexion either unilaterally or bilaterally, increase the height of the sitting surface so that the pelvis is able to move anteriorly over the femurs (to allow the creation of a neutral lordosis in the lumbar spine).

Therapist position: Standing or kneeling beside the patient. Hand position will depend on which levels of the spine need a change of curvature (see verbal/manual cues). Correct the thoracic curve first, then the lumbar curve, then the head/cervical position.

Therapist facilitation: Verbal cues
For areas of decreased thoracic kyphosis (usually accompanied by excessive erector spinae activity):

"Let the chest sink" or "go heavy under my hand"

"As your chest sinks, imagine your back opening between your shoulder blades"

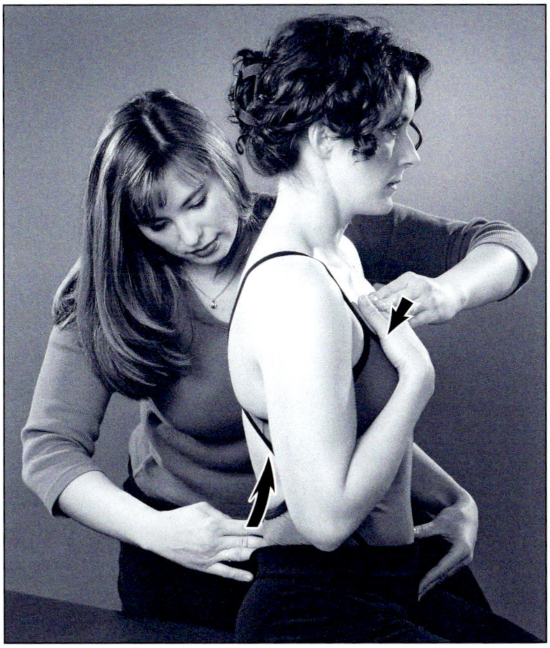

Figure 7.4 Neutral Spine: Sitting. Therapist points of control are the sternum and the lumbar spine. Patient points of control are the sternum and the superior pubic bone. The therapist's hand helps the patient create a "sinking" or "heaviness" on the sternum to facilitate an increase in thoracic kyphosis in the upper thoracic spine. The therapist's fingers at the lower lumbar spinous processes produce a gentle cranial and anterior pressure to facilitate a lifting of the sacrum, tilting of the pelvis forward, and gentle lumbar lordosis for levels of a flattened curve.

"Imagine that the distance from your sternum to your belly button is decreasing as you let the chest go heavy"

For areas of increased thoracic kyphosis:

"Imagine a string attached to your back (palpate at level of increased curve); the string is gently being pulled up to heaven"

"Imagine that your sternum is being gently lifted"

For a decreased lumbar lordosis (flexed lumbar spine):

"Imagine a string attached to your tailbone, and someone else is gently pulling the string up to heaven"

"Grow tall from the tailbone"

"Let your pelvis fall forward as you grow tall from my fingers"

"Let your buttocks go wide, let your hips fold"

"Allow the ball to roll underneath you as the pelvis falls forward"

Therapist facilitation:
Manual cues/Key points of control:
Options for therapist hand placement (points of control):

- Upper sternum (for loss of upper thoracic kyphosis)
- Lower sternum (for loss of lower thoracic kyphosis)
- Posterior thorax/rib cage (for excessive thoracic kyphosis)
- Lumbar spine spinous processes (at level where more lordosis is required)
- Manubriosternal symphysis and superior pubic bone (to cue vertical alignment of these points)

Iliac crests and hip folds (to facilitate anterior pelvic tilt over hips)

As the verbal cues are given, the therapist uses the points of control to create the ideal curvatures. To facilitate increased thoracic kyphosis, the hand on the sternum creates an inferior and posterior pressure. To decrease an excessive kyphosis, the hands lift the rib cage from the sides or give a superior and slightly anterior pressure at the levels of excessive curve. To correct a flat lumbar spine, the fingers push gently anterior and superior, creating a "lifting" sensation. For an excessive lumbar lordosis at one or two segments, focus on facilitating a lordosis at levels above or below that are flexed, and then "lengthening" or "stretching" the curve at the hyperextended segment(s).

Ideal response: The creation of the lumbar lordosis should be a "release" into an optimum curve, not a forced effort with contraction of the erector spinae.

- As the lumbar lordosis occurs the sternal hand should not move superior or anterior (the thoracic kyphosis should be maintained).
- The goal is to create a gentle, even kyphosis in the thoracic spine, a gentle, even lordosis in the lumbar spine, and a gentle lordosis in the cervical spine (avoid having one or two segments excessively flexed or extended).
- The manubriosternal symphysis should be vertically in line with the pubic bone; body weight should be centered equally over the ischial tuberosities ("sitz bones").
- The erector spinae muscles should not be excessively active (palpate to check for hypertonicity).
- See Video Clip 7.5: The patient performs the first two postural adjustments incorrectly; the sternum lifts and the thoracic spine extends. The final two repetitions illustrate the correct maintenance of the thoracic kyphosis while creating a lordosis localized to the lumbar spine.

Progressions/Other considerations:

- Use the feeling of a pelvic rock forwards and backwards to help dissociate pelvic from thoracic motion, and to feel the place of body weight over the ischial tuberosities – if the pelvis is posteriorly tilted, the patient will feel their weight behind the ischial tuberosities; if the pelvis is anteriorly tilted, they will feel their weight in front of the ishcial tuberosities.
- The breath can be used to facilitate the proper curves as well – "breathe deeply and allow the air to fill the space:"
  - Between your shoulder blades (if midthorax is lordotic)
  - Beneath your sternum (if midthorax is kyphotic)
  - Between your lowest ribs
    - Posteriorly (if lordotic)
    - Anteriorly (if kyphotic)
- Once you have facilitated a neutral spine position, ask the patient to maintain the new position and breathe normally.
- Observe what happens to spinal position with breathing – apical breathing often causes excessive thoracolumbar extension; re-educate breathing pattern (lateral costal expansion) to facilitate maintenance of the neutral spine position.
- You can use theraband around the rib cage to give proprioceptive feedback for the optimal breathing pattern (especially effective to encourage posterolateral expansion and minimize thoracolumbar extension). See Video Clip 7.6.
- Once the neutral spine can be attained and maintained while breathing, add a conscious recruitment of the lumbopelvic and/or thoracic local stabilizers.

Correcting rotational/sidebending asymmetry (see Video Clip 7.6)
Once the spinal curves are corrected in the sagittal plane, corrections can be made to any rotation/sidebending faults. It is important to realize that the position of the scapula and altered activity or length/strength relationships of the scapulothoracic muscles can have a significant impact on the position and function of the thoracic spine.

Therapist Facilitation: Manual and Verbal Cues: Hands on the lateral aspect of the rib cage. Facilitate a "lift" and "lengthening" of the rib cage on the side of the sidebending concavity. Give left or right lateral pressure to correct a shift. Use wiggling of the thorax to release excessive activity in the global muscles (to release bracing) and allow you to move and support the thorax into an optimal position.

- One hand under scapula, one hand on iliac crest; ask the patient to "Imagine that the distance between my hands is lengthening", "open the space between my hands."
- Encircle the rib cage with one arm and use the other hand to support the side closest to you. Provide gentle traction ("Let me support your rib cage") and laterally translate/rotate the rib cage into a neutral position (See Video Clip 7.6).
- Ask the patient to maintain the new position and breathe normally (see considerations above).

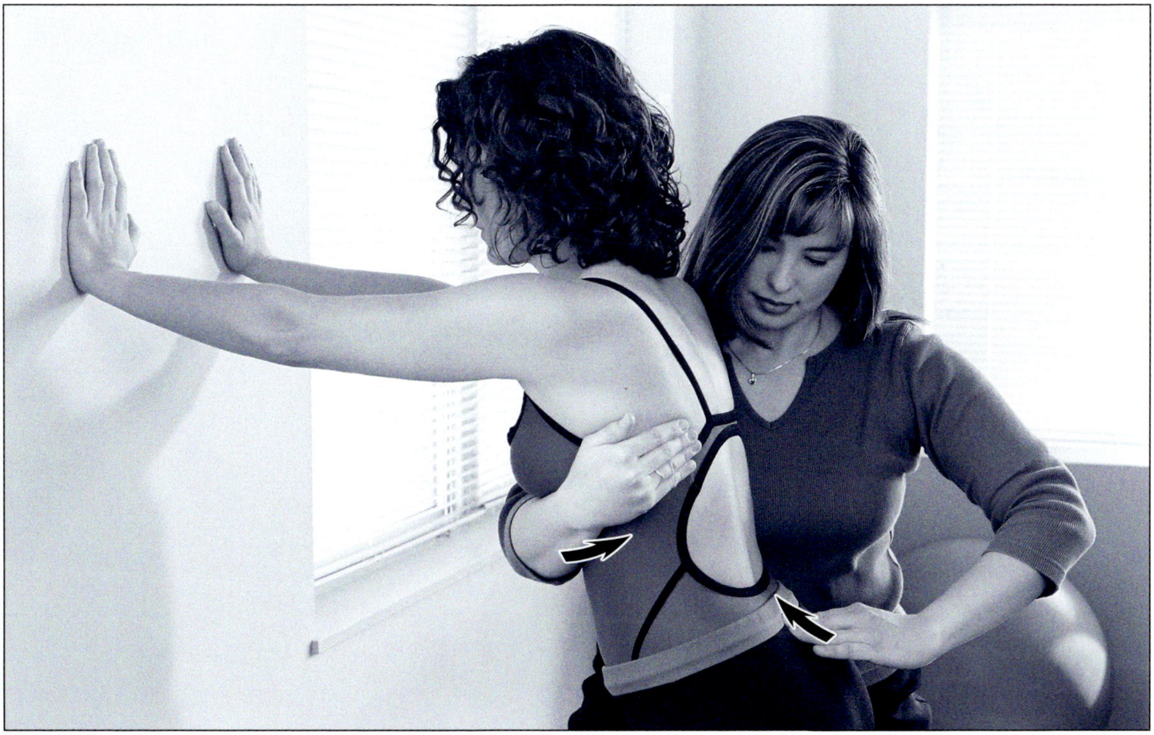

Figure 7.7 Neutral Spine: Standing Forward Lean on Wall. This is a useful position to train the ability of the thorax to transfer loads through a weight bearing upper extremity. Prior to adding arm movement, the patient must be able to attain and maintain control of a neutral spine position. In this example, the therapist uses one arm to support and gently traction the lower thorax. Subsequently, an inferior-posterior force is applied, thus facilitating an ideal thoracic kyphosis. The caudal hand provides a gentle cranial and anterior pressure to facilitate a lumbar lordosis in the flexed lumbar segments. Verbal cues are given concurrently with the manual facilitation.

These manual and verbal cues can be adapted to facilitate neutral spine in other positions such as supported standing, standing, and standing forward lean on wall (see Figure 7.7).

Four Point Kneeling (see Figure 7.8)

Patient position: 4 Point Kneeling on the floor or on a plinth; shoulders over hands, hips over knees. If there is a unilateral or bilateral restriction of hip flexion, the hips should be allowed to rock forward of the knees (otherwise the patient will be unable to attain a lumbar lordosis).

Therapist position: Kneeling or standing beside the patient. Hand placement will depend on the areas of thoracic and lumbar curvatures that need correction.

Therapist facilitation: Verbal cues

For decreased thoracic kyphosis:

"Let me have your rib cage; let your back open as I lift your chest"

"Take a breath and bring the air into your back"

For decreased lumbar lordosis:

"Let your buttocks go wide and the low back fall into a gentle arch"

"Keep your upper back open as you lengthen under my fingers"

"Stay supported and open in your rib cage as you let the pelvis fall forward towards the floor, letting the hips fold"

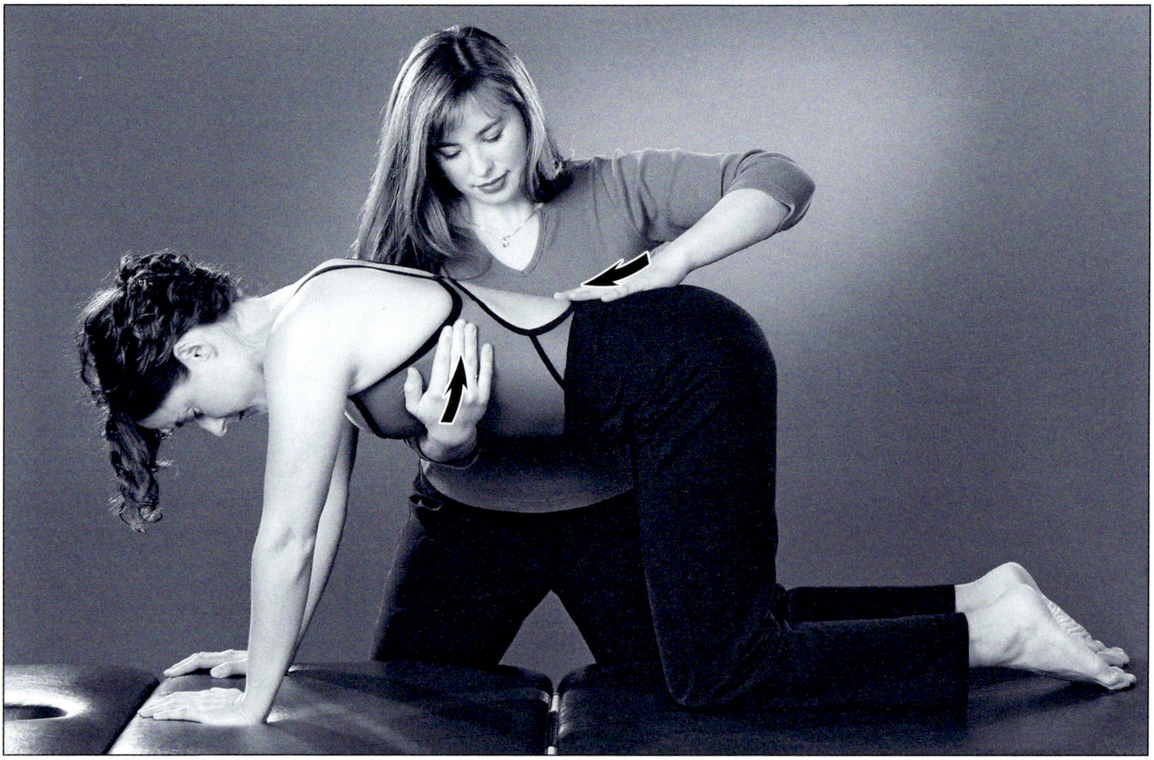

Figure 7.8 Neutral Spine: 4 Point Kneeling. This position is more challenging and a progression from the Standing Forward Lean on Wall position. Prior to adding arm or leg movement, the patient must be able to attain and maintain control of a neutral spine position. In this example the therapist uses the cranial arm under the rib cage to produce a thoracic kyphosis at the desired levels with a posterior force (lifting the rib cage). The caudal hand produces a cranial and anterior pressure in the lumbar segments to create a lordosis, while the verbal cues of lengthening through the low back, letting the buttocks go wide and releasing the hips are given.

For increased thoracic kyphosis:

"Lengthen your spine under my hands as you let your ribs fall to the floor"

For increased lumbar lordosis:

"Round out your back to the ceiling (reverse the curve into flexion), now let the low back arch again but think long and gentle (manual cueing is important here; see below).

Therapist facilitation:
Manual cues/Key points of control:

Options for therapist hand placement (points of control):

- Manubriosternal symphysis (for loss of upper thoracic kyphosis)
- Support under lower rib cage (for loss of lower thoracic kyphosis)
- Posterior thorax along spine (for excessive thoracic kyphosis)
- Lumbar spine spinous processes (at level where more lordosis is required or where curve needs lengthening)
- Iliac crests (to facilitate more even lumbar lordosis/lengthening through spine, anterior pelvic tilt over hips)
- Hip creases (to facilitate hip folding and widening of buttocks)

As the verbal cues are given, the therapist uses the points of control to create the ideal curvatures. To facilitate increased thoracic kyphosis, fingers under the sternum can press gently posteriorly (up to the ceiling), or the whole arm can support the rib cage and lift it posteriorly to open up the posterior thorax. To decrease an excessive kyphosis, one hand on the posterior thorax produces an anterior and slightly cranial pressure while a hand on the sacrum provides an inferior distraction to create a sensation of "lengthening" to go with the verbal cue. To correct a flat lumbar spine, the fingers push gently anterior and superior, creating a "lengthening" sensation as the pelvis falls forward but the thoracic spine stays supported into a neutral kyphosis. For an excessive lumbar lordosis at one or two segments, have the patient reverse the entire lumbar curve into flexion, then focus on facilitating a lordosis at levels above or below that are flexed as the patient returns into a lordosis. Use a light "wiggle" through the iliac crests with a caudal pull to create the sensation of "lengthening" or "stretching" the curve at the hyperextended segment(s). Head and neck position is corrected after releasing the support for the trunk.

Ideal response: As you release your manual support, the patient should be able to maintain the new position of gentle thoracic kyphosis and lumbar lordosis, without excessive bracing with the abdominals or breath holding. Ask the patient to maintain the position and breathe normally. If there is an anterior collapse of the upper thorax, loss of control through the scapulae, loss of the lumbar lordosis, or bracing and breath holding (the entire trunk becomes stiff), the patient is not ready for exercises in this position. The Standing Forward Lean on Wall position should be used first.

Progressions/Other Considerations:

- Have patient breathe in, breathe out, then gently connect to the deep lumbo-pelvic stabilizers. Gradually release your support as you ask the patient to hold that position.
- As the patient to come out of the position into kneeling. Go back into 4 point kneel and see if the patient can find the optimal position on their own. Repeat the manual/verbal cueing as needed, but reduce the manual support to train the patient to find the correct position on their own.
- Rotational/sidebending asymmetries can be corrected in this position using cues as described above in sitting.

Isolation of the local thoracic segmental stabilizers

Patient position: Facilitation of the thoracic segmental stabilizers can be done in any position; generally it is easiest to minimize excessive global activity in more supported positions (prone); once a confident contraction is attained in these positions then more upright and functional positions can be used as a progression. Since the prone position is used to assess the muscle bulk (see Figure 4.32, Video Clip 4.32), it can be the first position used to teach isolation of the segmental stabilizers. If the patient has difficulty in this position, sitting (in neutral spine) may be easier, due to the increased proprioceptive and afferent input that an upright, weight bearing position provides.

Prone: ensure that the thorax is supported into as neutral a position as possible and that there is relaxation of the thoracic erector spinae. If there is a lordosis in the thorax, a rolled towel can be placed vertically under the sternum to passively support the thorax into kyphosis. Arms should be relaxed at the sides or over the edge of the bed. Arms overhead should be avoided as this can alter spinal position if the latissimus dorsi muscle is tight, and can also increase erector spinae tone.

Sitting: use the techniques described above to help the patient find neutral spine. The patient should be sitting on a firm surface with the arms relaxed and hands resting on the thighs. If the patient has great difficulty attaining or maintaining neutral spine in sitting it will not be a good position to facilitate the thoracic segmental stabilizers and an alternate position such as prone should be used.

Therapist position: Standing beside the patient, palpate bilaterally and close to the spinous processes at the level you want to facilitate. One hand will facilitate the segmental contraction by letting the fingers or thumbs sink into the muscle (providing tactile and proprioceptive input) while the verbal commands are given. The other hand will palpate at one of four places to help create the image being used:

- In prone or sitting, palpate just medial and inferior to the ASIS (where you palpate transversus abdominis) on one side. If the

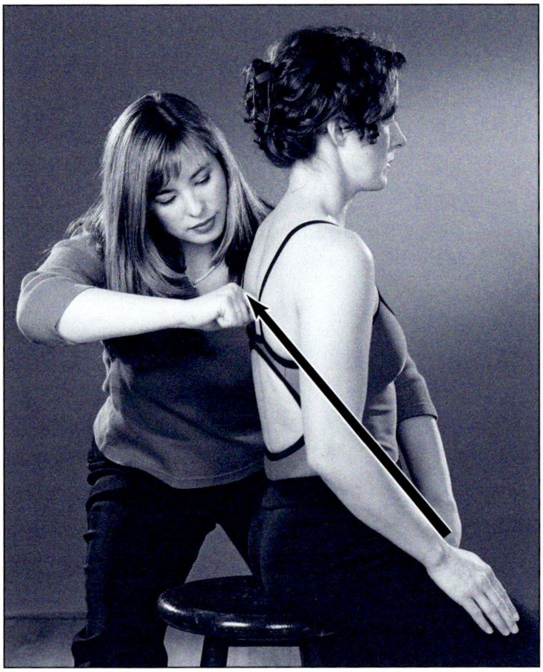

Figure 7.9 Isolation of Thoracic Segmental Stabilizers: Sitting. The height of the stool allows the patient to attain a neutral lumbopelvic position when there is a restriction of hip flexion range of motion. The therapist palpates and sinks the finger and thumb bilaterally into the segmental stabilizing muscles at one thoracic level. The other hand applies bilateral pressure in the upper inner thigh with the thumb and first finger. Deepening pressure is applied at these points sequentially as the patient is given an image of connecting a guy wire to suspend the spine. "Breathe in, then breathe out. Slowly, gently imagine you are connecting a wire that is starting from here (give pressure at the inner thighs), coming up and through your body, and connecting to my fingers here in your spine (give anterior and cranial pressure at the thoracic segment)". If the image is effective for the patient, you will feel a slow development of tension in the segmental muscle. Assess for symmetry between the right and left sides. (The arrow indicates the image of the wire.)

patient is sitting, a bilateral palpation can be achieved by spreading your hand such that your thumb sinks into one side and your fourth or fifth finger sinks into the other.

- In prone or sitting, palpate between the upper inner thigh (bilateral pressure) (see Figure 7.9).
- In sitting, palpate just superior to the pubic bone.
- In prone or sitting, palpate in the mid-axillary line, at the rib correlating to the level of the segmental muscle that you are trying to isolate (palpate at the side of less bulk) (see Figure 7.10).

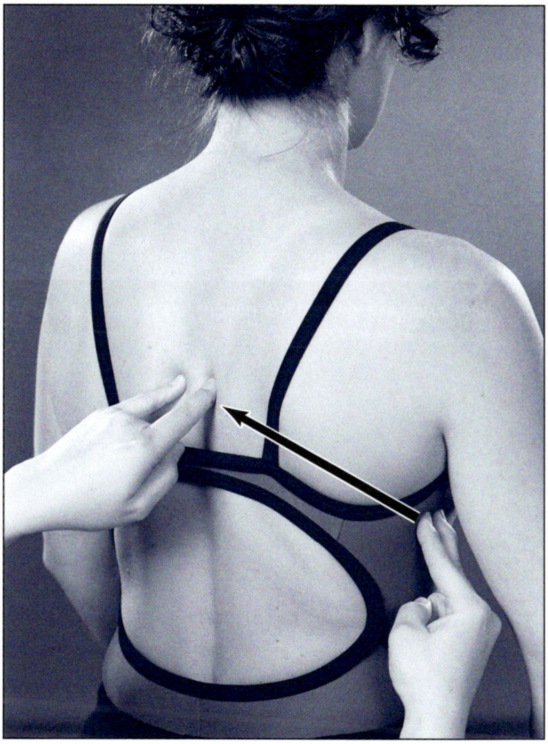

Figure 7.10 Isolation of Thoracic Segmental Stabilizers: Sitting. The therapist facilitates the image of drawing the ribs into the spine by palpating in the mid-axillary line. The fingers of the other hand sink into the segmental muscles at one thoracic level. As you give the verbal cues, apply sequential pressure, first in the mid-axillary line, then at the thoracic segment. "Breathe in, breathe out. Now slowly, lightly connect a line from your rib here (pressure in mid-axillary line), to my fingers in your spine here (pressure at thoracic segment)."

Therapist facilitation: Verbal cues

The image of supporting tent-wires, guy-wires, or connecting strings is used in all of these images (see Figure 7.11). The point of palpation of the segmental muscle is the consistent feature, and this is where the guy-wires are imaged to be attached to. The varying factor is where the initiation of the connection starts (the different palpation points above); choose the point that produces the best contraction of the segmental muscle. The image is created verbally with these instructions:

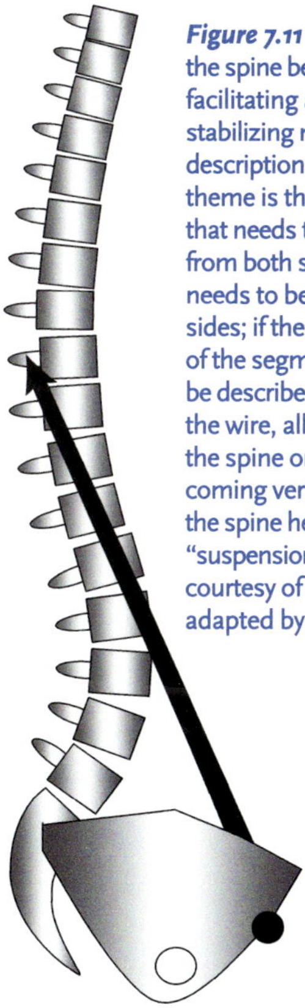

Figure 7.11 Images that create the feeling of the spine being "suspended" are effective for facilitating a connection to the deep stabilizing muscles of the spine. Various descriptions can be used, but the common theme is that the spine is a central pole that needs to be supported by tension wires from both sides. The tension in the wires needs to be equal on the right and left sides; if there is a loss of activity in one side of the segmental stabilizing muscles it can be described as a loss of the connection in the wire, allowing rotation and collapse of the spine on that side. The idea of energy coming vertically up the wires to support the spine helps to create the sense of "suspension". This figure is reproduced courtesy of Dr. Paul Hodges and was adapted by Lee L J for this text.

> "Imagine a tent wire that is going to suspend your spine, and it is starting from your pelvic floor (palpate at pubic bone) and slowly coming up and through your body to connect to the point where my fingers are in this muscle in your back."

> "Breathe in, breathe out, and connect your support wire from here (provide tactile cue at pubic bone or other point) to here (provide tactile cue at segmental muscle)".

For the palpation point in the mid-axillary line, a few different images can be used:

> "Imagine you are drawing the ribs into your spine"

> "Imagine the vertebra is a nut, and the ribs as a nutcracker. Think of drawing the ribs towards the vertebra and squeezing the nut"

> "Connect a line from my finger here to my finger here"

Manual cues/Key points of control: Provide slow, deepening pressure with your fingers as you help the patient create the image – the pressure is applied sequentially from the anterior/inferior point first then at the segmental muscle point posteriorly. At both points the pressure is slightly cranial to reinforce the feeling of the spine being suspended by the wire (tensegrity vs. compression).

Ideal response: A deep, tonic swelling of the segmental muscle, which is felt as a gradual increase in tension under your fingers (close to the spinous processes). You should sense that the contraction starts deeply and comes up into your fingers, as if the pads of your fingers are being indented, rather than the fingers being pushed off the back. Any rapid recruitment is indicative of a recruitment of the superficial muscles. With the rib cueing (mid-axillary line), be particularly observant for substitution with rhomboids and middle trapezius muscles. You should see no erector spinae or scapular muscle activity.

Progressions/Other considerations:

- Have the patient maintain the connection to the segmental muscle and breathe normally. Ensure an optimal breathing pattern.
- Watch for any recruitment of the global muscles (obliques, thoracic erector spinae, rectus abdominis, hip muscles, scapular muscles, sternocleidomastoid) and/or bracing of the rib cage which indicates excessive effort and recruitment of the dominant global muscles. Check for global rigidity by gentle "wiggling" the rib cage; if the rib cage is mobile then the global muscle system is not overactive.
- There should be no change in spinal orientation (maintain neutral spine) when the segmental muscles are recruited.
- The scapular muscles should remain relaxed (no scapular movement).
- If you palpate a co-contraction of transversus abdominis and/or the patient reports a feeling of lifting in the pelvic floor (submaximal) this is optimal as it is engaging the local stabilizers and a part of the normal low-load spinal support mechanism.
- The position of neutral spine is key in facilitating this muscle. Taping can be used to support a level of hypermobility or "give" or for proprioceptive feedback at desired levels.
- A significant alteration in the scapular resting position, especially a "dumped" scapula (depressed and downwardly rotated) can affect neutral thoracic position and make engaging the thoracic segmental stabilizers more difficult. To assess if this is a factor, manually support the scapula into a neutral position and repeat the

segmental muscle contraction facilitation. If it improves, use taping to support the scapula into a neutral position.

- Educate the patient on duration of holds, number of repetitions, and frequency of exercise. The goal is 10 second holds, 10 repetitions, with normal breathing. This will not be the starting point for the majority of patients. The key is to maintain an isolated contraction with breathing, and without substitution with global musculature. Your assessment of the patient's ability will guide your prescription (you may find that after 3 seconds of holding the patient starts to breath hold; you would then advise only 3 second holds, and then assess how many repetitions the patient can perform and maintain a good quality of contraction). The exercises should be practiced as frequently as possible to facilitate optimal motor learning; short sessions performed often throughout the day are preferred to one long session.
- As the patient is able to perform isolated segmental recruitment for longer durations and increasing repetitions, progress the exercise by moving from the initial supported positions to more functional, upright positions (sitting, supported standing, standing lean forward on wall). It is important to assess the ability of the patient to perform the isolated recruitment of the segmental muscles in each new position. Signs of excessive global muscle recruitment (eg. bracing) and change in breathing pattern are indications that the new position is too demanding and will direct the choice of position used. When introducing a new position, use the strategies described above for facilitating a neutral spine posture, then assess for isolation of the thoracic segmental stabilizers in the new position, and ensure that normal breathing can be maintained before adding limb movement or other global muscle progressions in that position.

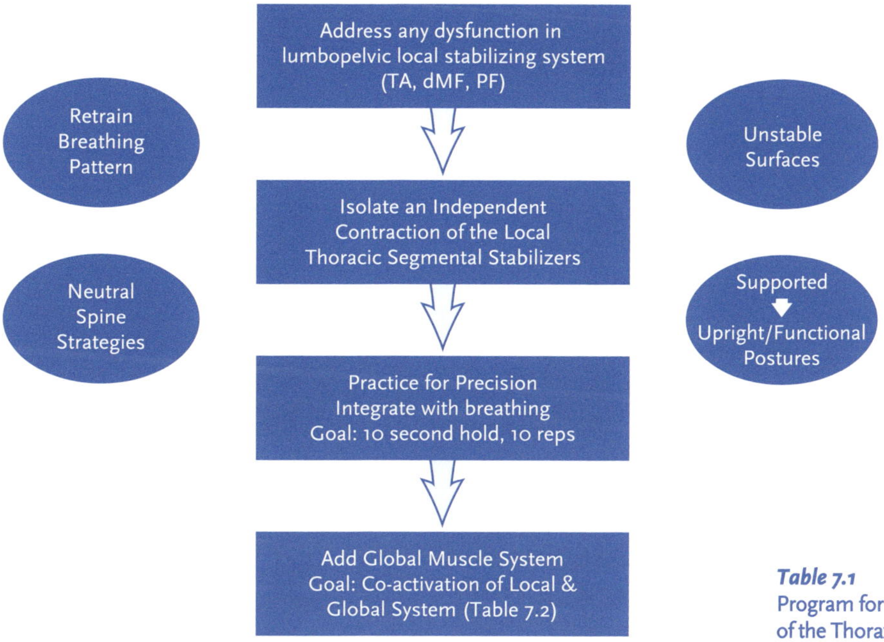

Table 7.1
Program for Stabilization of the Thorax

Exercise Progression – Adding the Global Muscles

Once the patient can isolate and hold a confident contraction of the thoracic segmental stabilizers at the dysfunctional segment without global muscle activity and with normal breathing, integration with the global muscles can be started. The goal is to maintain the co-contraction of the deep local system (thoracic segmental stabilizers, transversus abdominis, deep fibres of multifidus, pelvic floor) while maintaining positions and controlling movements that require low load global muscle activity. Care must be taken not to start global muscle exercises too early, and the ability to voluntarily isolate and tonically hold a segmental contraction should be reassessed often to ensure that control of the local system has not been lost. The specific exercise progression used will vary depending on each patient's presentation, but a general protocol for progression is presented in Tables 7.1 and 7.2. This protocol is adapted from the guidelines developed by Richardson et al (1999) for the lumbopelvic region.

General Principles (Table 7.3)

- "Connect first" – teach the patient to perform a pre-contraction of the thoracic segmental stabilizers as the starting point for each exercise.
- Palpate and monitor the segmental muscle recruitment and control of joint position during the exercises, especially when adding a new progression. Ensure that the muscle does not turn off and that there are no signs of loss of control into the direction of hypermobility.
- Focus on low load and control of movement.
- Use the "Manual Cues/Key Points of Control" described above for attaining neutral spine and isolating the segmental stabilizers to provide tactile feedback and assist control at the levels where segmental hypermobility or multisegmental collapse occurs during the exercise movements.
- Avoid fast ballistic movements.
- Progress from stable to unstable surfaces to increase proprioceptive input and challenge.
- Check for excessive global muscle activity by monitoring breathing pattern (should continue to see lateral costal and abdominal expansion) and by monitoring for bracing/rigidity.
- Incorporate local muscle co-contraction into daily functional activities as early and as often as possible; break down functional tasks into component movements and use separate components as an exercise.

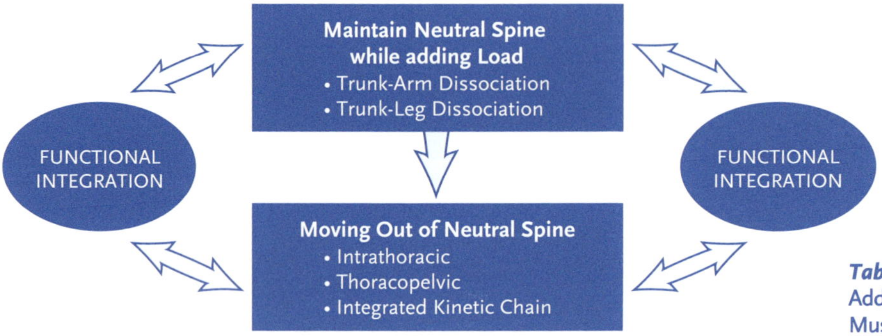

Table 7.2 Adding the Global Muscle System

General Principles for Progression: Adding the Global Muscles

- "Connect first": instruct the patient to pre-contract the thoracic segmental stabilizing muscles.
- Palpate and monitor the maintenance of tonic recruitment of the deep segmental muscles throughout the exercise.
- Focus on low load and control of movement.
- Use "Key Points of Control" to provide tactile feedback and assist control at the levels where segmental hypermobility or multisegmental collapse occurs.
- Avoid fast ballistic movements.
- Progress from stable to unstable surfaces to increase proprioceptive input and challenge.
- Monitor breathing pattern and avoid bracing/rigidity.
- Incorporate local muscle co-contraction into daily functional activities as early and as often as possible.
- Focus on co-contraction and control of position instead of single muscle strengthening.
- Upper/middle thoracic dysfunction: ensure integration with arm movements; middle/lower thoracic dysfunction: ensure integration with leg movements; many functional activities require integration of whole kinetic chain.
- If high load and high speed activities are required, add at end stages. Continue with concurrent low load exercises.
- Design exercise progressions based on individual patient presentation and functional requirements.

Table 7.3

- Focus on co-contraction and control of position instead of single muscle strengthening.
- For upper and middle thoracic control integration with arm movements is key; for middle and lower thoracic control integration with leg movements is key. Many sport specific and work activities require integration of the whole kinetic chain.
- If high load and high speed activities are required for work or sport, add these at end stages and ensure that low load, slow speed control is present for the same movement pattern first. High speed/high load activities should be only one part of the patient's exercise program; low load exercises should be continued concurrently to ensure continued function of the local system.
- There are many variations and options possible for each of the following categories. For each section, several progressions are presented, but the reader is encouraged to use the principles and guidelines in this chapter to guide the creation of other exercise progressions that may be necessary for a specific patient presentation.

Maintaining neutral spine while adding load

The goal for all exercises in this section is to maintain a local system co-contraction in a neutral spine position against the challenge of limb loading. The spinal curves should be monitored and the relationship between the lumbopelvic region and the thorax should be maintained throughout the exercise. The movements should be slow and controlled in both the concentric and eccentric phases of movement.

Trunk-Arm Dissociation

1) Supine

Patient position: Crook lying in neutral spine on a flat surface; can progress to lying on a 1/2 roll or other unsupported surface. Arms are flexed to 90° so that the hands are vertically over the shoulder joints.

Exercise instruction: Cue the image that facilitates the contraction of the thoracic segmental stabilizers at the dysfunctional level, then cue breathing. Ask the patient to keep the spine still and the chest heavy as they move the arms into elevation through flexion.

Progressions/Other considerations:

- Progress from bilateral to unilateral movements of the arms. Bilateral movements will provide more challenge to flexion/extension control in the thorax, while unilateral movements will provide challenge to rotational control.
- Other options include arm abduction (see Figure 7.12) and arm extension (from 90° flexion down to the bed; can progress to past neutral over the edge of the bed).
- Add light weights (one to five pounds) in the hands to increase challenge.

2) Sitting

Patient position: Sitting on a firm surface, feet on the floor, in neutral spine.

Exercise instruction: Cue the image that facilitates the contraction of the segmental thoracic stabilizers, then cue breathing. Ask the patient to maintain the spinal position and the connection to the image while moving the arms into flexion, abduction, extension, or diagonal flexion/extension patterns.

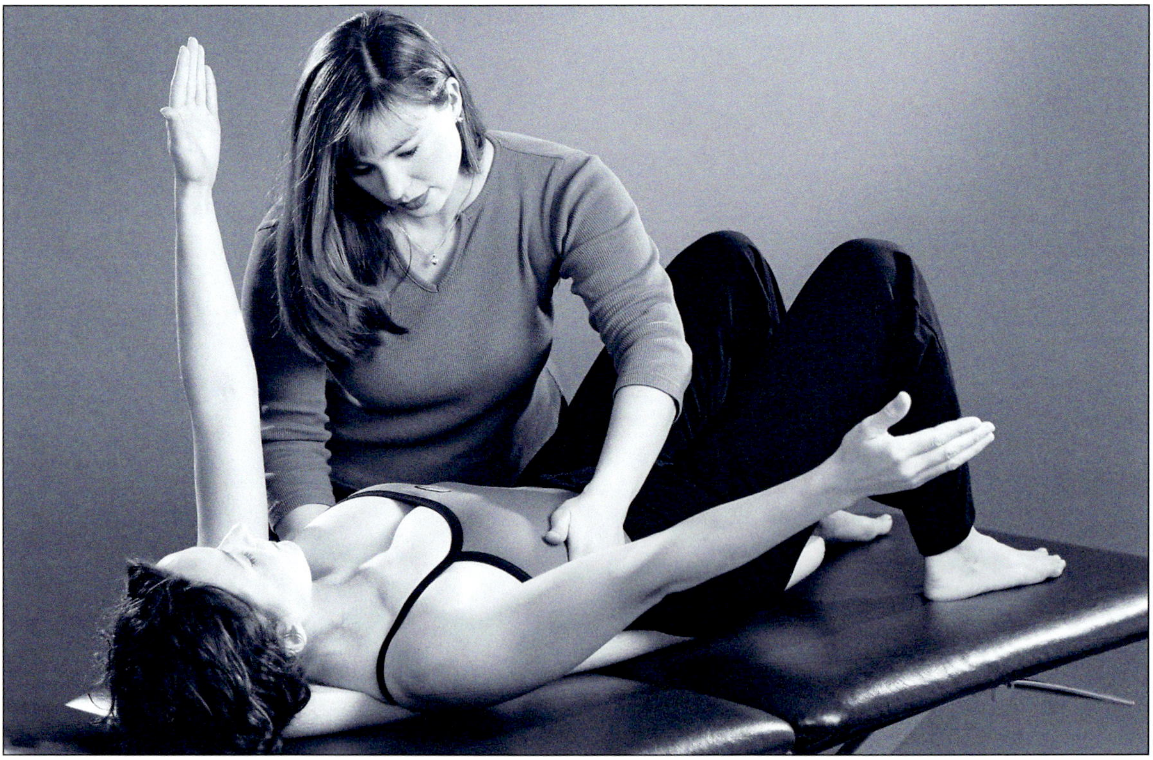

Figure 7.12 Maintaining Neutral Spine while adding Load: Trunk-Arm Dissociation. Supine.
The therapist monitors control of lateral shift at the rib cage and observes for rotation of the thorax as the patient moves the right arm into abduction.

Progressions/Other Considerations:

- Progress to sitting on a ball and/or feet on sissels.
- Start with no resistance, then progress to theraband resistance.
- Pull down motions require flexion control of the thorax, pull up motions require extension control, and unilateral or diagonal motions require rotational control.
- Examples:
  - Video Clip 7.13: The patient is sitting on a ball with a starting position of thoracic lordosis (loss of normal kyphosis). The therapist manually facilitates a neutral spine position, and then cues recruitment of the thoracic segmental stabilizers. When the contraction is felt the rib cage is gently rocked side to side to check for rigidity. The thoracic segmental muscles are then monitored for tonic contraction during the arm movement. The patient starts with bilateral pull downs then demonstrates a progression of the exercise to unilateral pull downs.
  - Video Clip 7.14 The patient is sitting on a ball with the thoracic spine in a starting position of right side bending and left lateral shift. The therapist manually facilitates a neutral spine position by correcting the right side bend and extension. The patient connects to the local stabilizers and then pulls the arm into a diagonal flexion pattern. The therapist continues to provide feedback to prevent collapse of the thorax into right sidebending during the exercise.

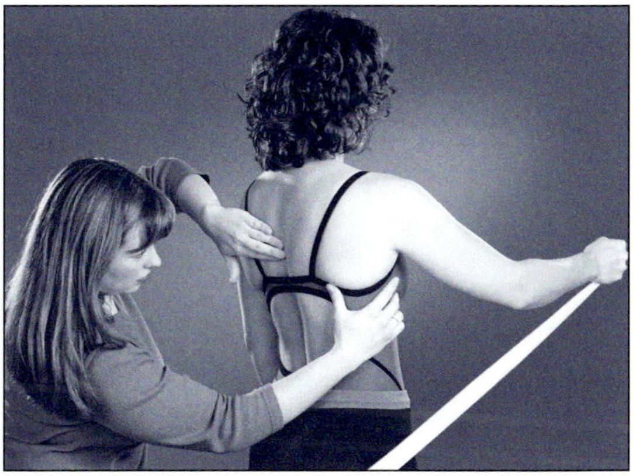

Figure 7.15 Maintaining Neutral Spine while adding Load: Trunk-Arm Dissociation. Standing.
The patient stands in neutral spine with weight equal on both feet. The segmental stabilizing muscles are recruited prior to moving the arm. In this example the therapist is facilitating the right thoracic segmental muscles while cueing control of the scapula during unilateral arm flexion against theraband resistance.

3) Supported Standing/ Standing
The same arm movements described above for the sitting position can be used in supported standing (with the back against a wall) or standing (see Figure 7.15). To challenge the base of support further, change the position of the feet to a lunge stance, then to standing on one leg, while maintaining neutral spinal alignment and performing the arm movements.

4) Prone on Ball (Figure 7.16)
Patient position: Kneeling prone over a ball with the thorax positioned so that the curve of the ball facilitates maintenance of the neutral thoracic kyphosis. If additional support in the thoracic curve is needed (for excessively lordotic curves) a towel roll can be placed vertically under the sternum.

Exercise instruction: Cue the image that facilitates the contraction of the thoracic segmental stabilizers at the dysfunctional level, then cue breathing. Ask the patient to keep the thorax open and the lumbar spine lengthened as the arm is lifted off the ball.

Progressions/Other considerations: As a progression to both Trunk-Arm Dissociation and Trunk-Leg Dissociation (see below), add an opposite leg extension to the arm lift. Start

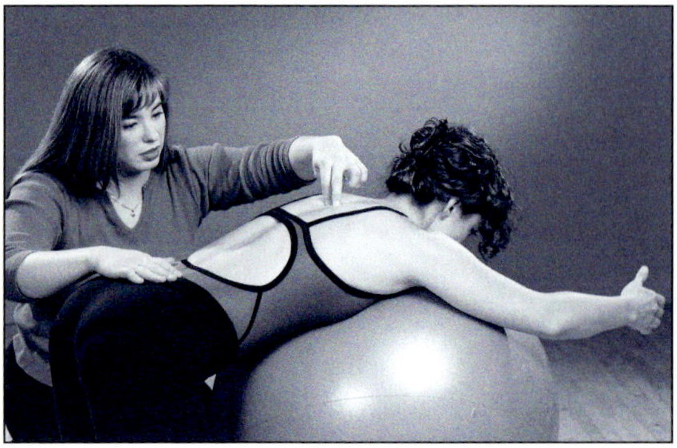

Figure 7.16 Maintaining Neutral Spine while adding Load: Trunk-Arm Dissociation. Prone over Ball. The therapist provides feedback at the thoracic segmental stabilizing muscles to facilitate a tonic contraction while gently cueing control of the lumbar lordosis as the patient slowly lifts the arm. The arm does not have to move through a large range of motion but the neutral spine position and the local muscle contraction needs to be maintained throughout the exercise. The therapist observes for any extension, rotation, or lateral shifts in the thoracic segment as the arm is lifted.

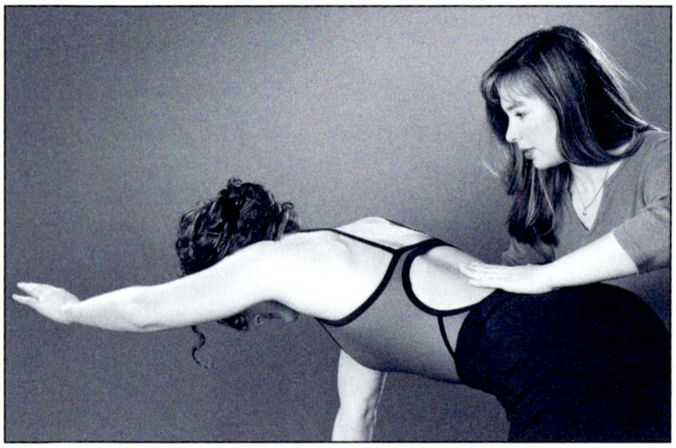

Figure 7.18 Maintaining Neutral Spine while adding Load: Trunk-Arm Dissociation. Upper Extremity Weight Bearing in Four Point Kneeling. The therapist's cranial hand provides tactile feedback under the upper sternum to cue the thoracic kyphosis while the caudal hand cues the maintenance of the lumbar lordosis. The levels of poor control are observed for aberrant movements as the patient lifts the arm from the floor.

with a small range of motion and ensure control of the neutral spine before progressing to larger ranges of motion.

5) Upper Extremity Weight Bearing (Closed Kinetic Chain)

Patient position: The Standing Forward Lean on Wall position is the starting position for training load transfer through a weight bearing upper extremity.

Exercise instruction: The therapist facilitates a neutral spine position and then cues the segmental muscle contraction. Start with bilateral control by instructing the patient to perform a push up action; ask the patient to keep the thorax still (no collapsing into extension) and let the movement occur as a hinge from the feet so that the spine stays connected as one unit.

Progressions/Other considerations:

- Progress to rotational control with a one arm lift from the wall: see Video Clip 7.17.

In this video clip, the patient first performs three left arm lifts with poor technique. The starting position is a lordotic and right side bent thorax. As the left arm is lifted, extension of the thorax increases and a rotation occurs. The therapist then corrects the starting position to a neutral spine position, cues a segmental muscle contraction to control the level of dysfunction, then has the patient repeat the arm lift with no spinal movement.

- Progress from the wall to Four Point Kneeling; see Figure 7.18.
- For the one arm lift, start with the hands placed close together (narrow), then progress to hands wider apart.
- If the exercises can not be controlled in the Standing Forward Lean on Wall position, do not progress to Four Point Kneeling.

6) Functional Integration

The patient can be made aware of controlling neutral spine position during activities such as reaching for and pushing objects with the arms. Choose activities that are most relevant to the patient's work and sport requirements. Simulation of these activities can be performed in the clinic to reinforce appropriate patterning and control.

Trunk-Leg Dissociation

1) Supine

   Leg loading exercises and their progressions have been described as exercises to train lumbopelvic control (Lee 2001, Richardson et al, 1999, Sahrmann 2001); examples include heel slides, bent knee fall-outs, and one leg alternating leg lifts performed from the start position of crook lying. These exercises can be challenging for patients with thoracic dysfunction, especially when the dysfunction is in the middle to lower thoracic regions. Compensatory shifts and loss of control of the neutral spine position can be observed. For a description of these exercises the reader is referred to the above sources. The key to applying these exercises to thoracic stabilization is the focus on thoracic segmental control and maintaining the correct relationship between the lumbopelvis and thorax (neutral spine) during leg movements.

2) Sitting

   In this position Trunk-Leg Dissociation exercises can focus on either a) movement of the trunk on the hips or b) movement of the legs under the trunk.

   a) Sitting lean forward (see Video Clip 7.19)

      Patient Position: Sitting on the edge of a plinth, chair, or ball. If there is a restriction of hip flexion range of motion the surface should be high enough to allow the pelvis to flex over the femoral heads. The feet are supported on the floor.

      Exercise instruction: Cue a neutral spine position; then place the patient's hands in the anterior hip creases. Have the patient "connect" to the local system, then instruct the patient to hinge at the hips to bring the trunk forward over the hips while keeping the spine still. Only allow movement through a range of motion where there is no loss of neutral spine. Start with small amounts of movement and progress to larger ranges. This exercise can be progressed to standing (Sahrmann's "Waiter's Bow" (2001)).

   b) Hip flexion or knee extension

      Patient position: Sitting in neutral spine, feet supported on the floor; exercise can be progressed to sitting on a ball or other unstable surface.

      Exercise instruction: "Connect to the thoracic segmental stabilizers, then slowly lift one knee up and fold at the hip (hip flexion) as you keep the spine still." Or, ask the patient to straighten the knee while keeping the spine still.

3) Supported Standing (see Figure 7.20)

   Patient position: Standing in neutral spine against a ball on the wall. The ball should be placed such that it supports the lumbar lordosis and does not restrict the movement of the thorax into a neutral kyphosis. The hips should be in neutral rotation, the knees under the hips, the second toe of each foot in line with the middle of the patella, with equal body weight distributed over each foot.

   Exercise instruction: Advise the patient that movement is only to occur in the legs; the spine stays still and suspended by the "guy wires". The patient is asked to squat "as if sitting in a chair", flexing at the hips, knees and ankles, while maintaining the neutral spine position.

   Progressions/Other considerations: Progressions can include: lunge position (see Figure 7.21), lunge then knee lift (posterior leg lifts up into hip flexion), squat on wobble board, one leg squat.

4) Upper Extremity Weight Bearing (Closed Kinetic Chain)
Patient positioning and cueing is the same as for Trunk-Arm Dissociation (prone on ball, four point kneeling), but the exercise movement involves lifting one leg at a time into extension or diagonal extension movements.

5) Standing: Rotation Control (see Video Clip 7.22)
Patient position: Standing in neutral spine, in stance position with the legs, back leg is up on the ball of the foot. Weight is focused on the front leg. Knee remains facing anterior, middle of the patella is over the second toe and in line with the hip joint.

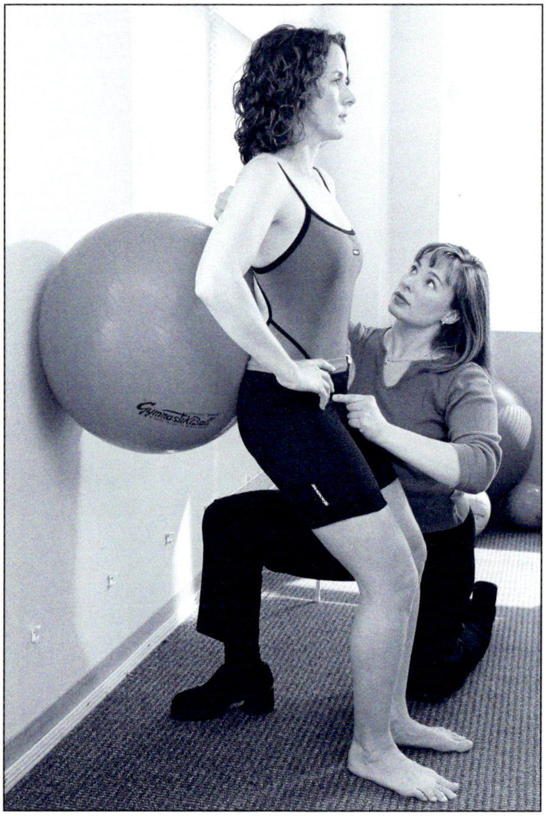

Figure 7.20 Maintaining Neutral Spine while adding Load: Trunk-Leg Dissociation. Squat in Supported Standing. The therapist is bilaterally palpating medial to the ASIS's and cueing a guy-wire image up to the thoracic segmental stabilizers in the mid-thoracic spine. The patient performs a squat as the therapist monitors the neutral spine position and segmental thoracic contraction. There should be no change in the thoracic or lumbopelvic position as the hips and knees are flexing.

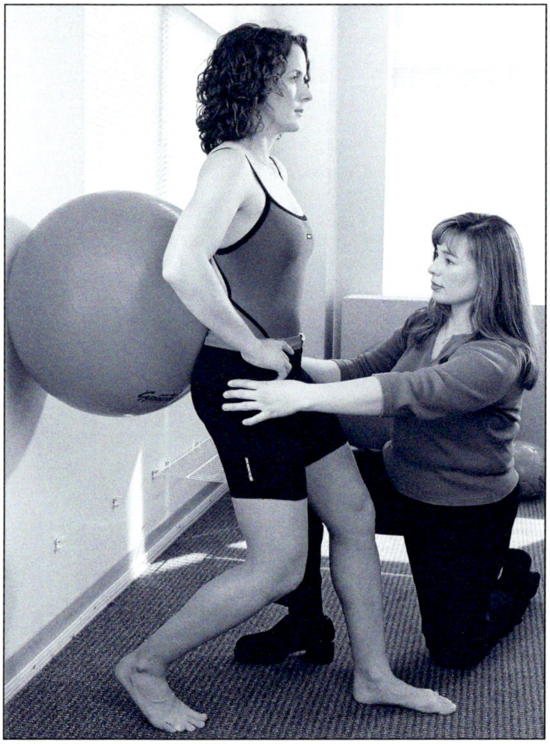

Figure 7.21 Maintaining Neutral Spine while adding Load: Trunk-Leg Dissociation. Lunge in Supported Standing. Changing the base of support is a progression of the squat exercise. The patient's body weight is distributed equally over both legs, with the posterior leg supported up on the ball of the foot. The deep local stabilizing muscles are recruited prior to the lunge movement; in this example the therapist provides tactile feedback at the anterior hip creases to facilitate folding (flexion) of the hips equally and maintenance of pelvic position during the movement. The thorax is observed for areas of loss of control and manual feedback provided as needed. Further challenge can be added by having the patient stand on 'sissels' or other unstable surfaces.

Exercise instruction: Cue lumbopelvic and segmental thoracic local muscle recruitment, and instruct the patient to keep the leg still and the knee forward while rotating the pelvis and trunk as one unit over the leg (spin pelvis over femoral head). Cue the initiation of the rotation movement coming from just inside the ASIS.

Progressions/Other considerations: Do not allow any lateral or posterior pelvic tilting as the pelvis rotates. Monitor the knee and give tactile cueing to keep the knee facing forward. Monitor the thoracic level of poor control, specifically watching for rotation and/or sidebending. Progress to performing the exercise while weight bearing only on the front leg.

6) Functional Integration
There are many options for progression in this category; a few examples are listed here. Again, the key is the maintenance of a neutral spine position; observe for any loss of thoracic position, lumbopelvic position, and the relationship of the thorax over the pelvis. Throughout the movements the spine should be "suspended" and "still" but not braced. Exercise examples:

a) Sit to Stand from chair or ball.

b) Forward Lunge against Unilateral theraband resistance (see Video Clip 7.23): The patient performs a forward lunge with the left leg with light resistance around the right shoulder from behind. The first three repetitions demonstrate a loss of thoracic control, with the thorax collapsing into right rotation and right sidebending. The therapist provides manual correction into neutral spine; the last three repetitions are performed correctly maintaining thoracic control. The theraband resistance can be placed on the ipsilateral or contralateral shoulder.

c) Step Up/Step Down (see Video Clip 7.24): The patient performs a step up with the left leg; note the right side bending and extension occurring in the T7 area during the first three repetitions. The therapist cues an awareness of the area of poor control by facilitating an "opening" on the right side; continued tactile feedback prevents the right sidebending as the exercise is repeated.

Moving out of neutral spine

Control of movements out of neutral spine is essential for stability during many functional activities. The therapist must carefully monitor the intersegmental relationships during these movements to ensure that there is equal movement and loading occurring at each segment and from each component in the kinetic chain of movement. For functional load transfer, the hypermobile segment(s) must be controlled during Intrathoracic movements out of neutral, during changes in Thoracopelvic orientation, and as a component part of an Integrated Functional Kinetic Chain.

Intrathoracic

Focus on retraining the movement where the directional hypermobility is most poorly controlled. Controlled segmental flexion, extension, rotation, sidebending, and combined movements are necessary for normal function. Start in more supported positions (sitting) and progress to kneeling, then standing, incorporating unstable surfaces whenever appropriate. Some examples of exercises in this category include:

1) Sitting: Cervical and Thoracic flexion and Return to Neutral Spine (see Video Clip 7.25): The patient starts in a position of neutral spine, using the local stabilizing system to maintain this start position. The therapist cues segmental cervical flexion, continuing down into the thoracic spine. Tactile feedback is provided along the spinous processes. Once the desired amount of flexion has occurred, cue a segmental return to neutral spine, avoiding bracing with

the global musculature of the thorax or neck. Progress by asking the patient to perform the exercise with the eyes closed.

2) Video Clip 7.26 Standing Pure Rotation and Combined Rotation with Flexion (this exercise should be first accomplished in sitting): The therapist cues a neutral spine position and connection to the segmental stabilizers. Theraband around the left shoulder provides resistance to right thoracic rotation; the therapist cues a pure rotation while providing feedback at the iliac crests to maintain a still pelvis. A progression is to add segmental flexion with the rotation. To add further challenge, the upper extremity is added to the chain of movement. This progression is shown in sitting in Figure 7.27. The therapist is providing tactile feedback to help the patient stay connected to the thoracic segmental stabilizers while the patient performs a PNF flexion pattern with the left arm along with right rotation and flexion. Use of the ball increases proprioceptive demand. Figure 7.28 illustrates further increasing complexity by progressing to standing; in this example an arm extension PNF pattern combined with thoracic rotation and extension is shown. Each component of the chain must be monitored for control (thoracic segment, thorax moving over stable pelvis/lower extremity, scapular movement on thorax, arm movement with scapula.

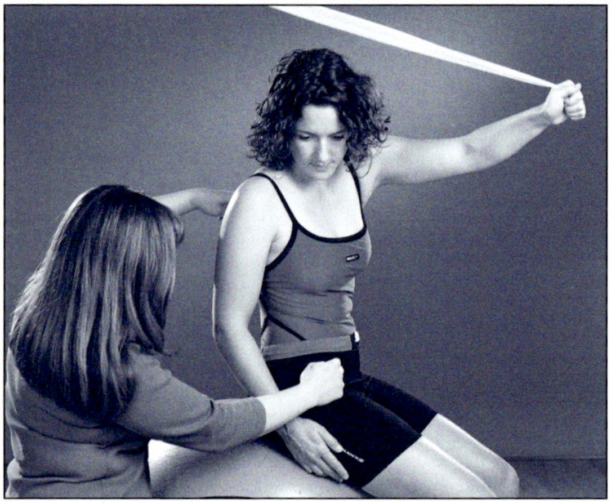

Figure 7.27 Moving out of Neutral Spine: Intrathoracic. Combined segmental rotation and flexion with upper extremity integration. The therapist is providing tactile facilitation of the 'guy-wire' image for the right side (the side of decreased thoracic segmental muscle recruitment). The patient performs a flexion PNF pattern with the left arm combined with right thoracic rotation and flexion. Prior to this exercise progression the patient should master control of right rotation in sitting, then right rotation and flexion.

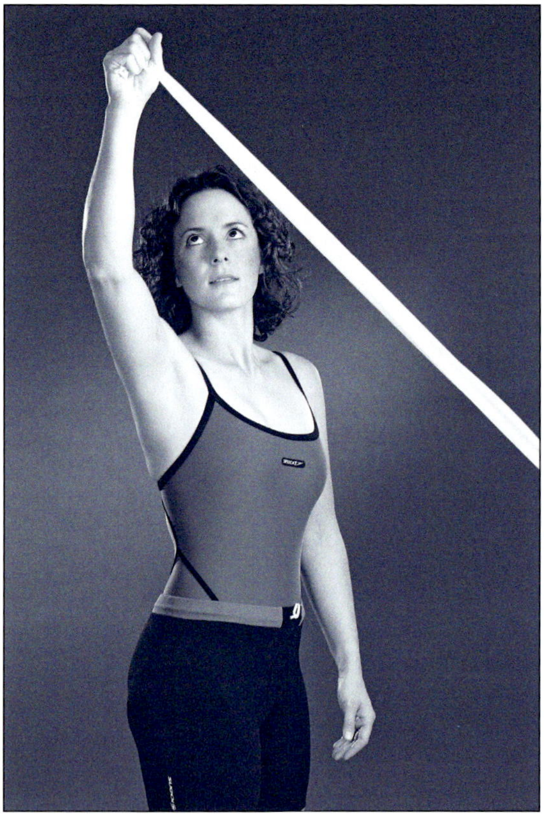

Figure 7.28 Moving out of Neutral Spine: Intrathoracic. Combined segmental rotation and extension with upper extremity integration. The patient has developed an internal sense of the images required to achieve recruitment of the thoracic local stabilizers and lumbopelvic local stabilizers to the point where manual facilitation from the therapist is no longer required. The starting position for the right hand is in front of the left hip. Prior to performing the movement, the patient thinks of "connecting", then moves the right arm in a diagonal extension PNF pattern while right rotating and extending the thorax. The pelvis remains still.

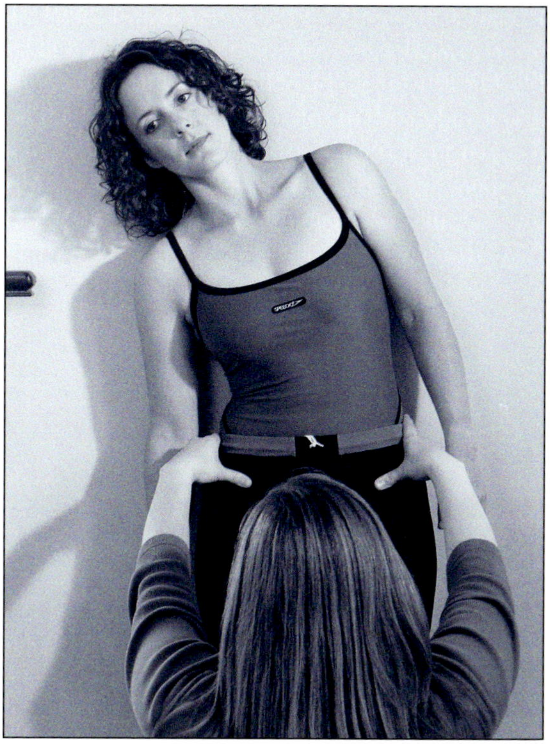

Figure 7.29 Moving out of Neutral Spine: Intrathoracic: Wall Side Bend. The patient stands against a wall to provide feedback; the goal is to achieve pure sidebending of the trunk without thoracic or pelvic rotation away from the wall. The therapist can provide tactile feedback to cue where the movement should occur and to prevent collapse, hinging, or rotation at a specific level. In this example the therapist monitors pelvic position.

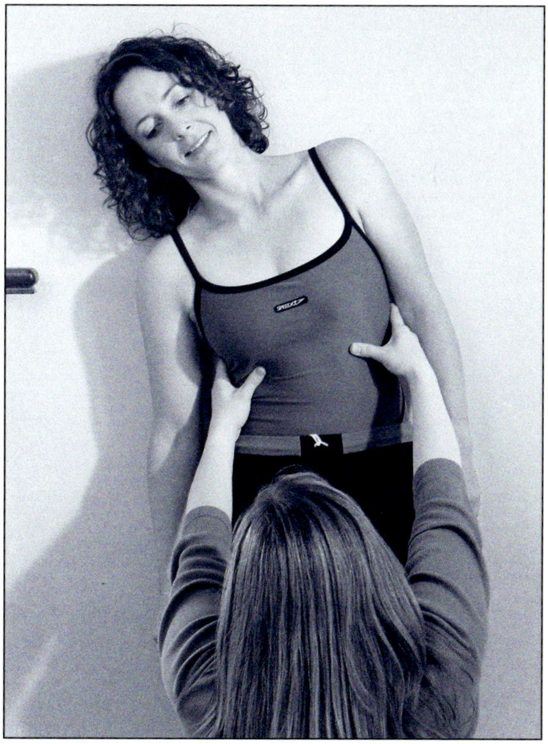

Figure 7.30 Moving out of Neutral Spine: Intrathoracic: Wall Side Bend. As the patient performs the side bending movement the therapist uses the ribcage to facilitate a pattern of segmental movement rather than hinging at one thoracic level.

3) Wall Side Bend (see Figures 7.29, 7.30): This exercise trains control of pure sidebending without segmental lateral shifting, hinging, or rotation. The wall provides tactile feedback so the patient can monitor if the pelvis or thorax rotates away from the wall. The therapist can add manual feedback at the rib cage or pelvis to encourage movement or control at desired levels.

Thoracopelvic

These exercises focus on training the ability to dissociate movement of the thorax from the pelvis and vice versa. The ability to control thoracopelvic movement is an essential requirement of many functional activities, from those as basic as walking to more complex sport maneuvers. These two exercises provide a starting point, but the principles can be applied to component movements of relevant functional activities (e.g. a golf swing) to produce a multitude of patient-specific exercise progressions.

1) Rowing Back (see Video Clip 7.31): the patient starts sitting with the knees bent on a plinth or the floor. Place a small ball between the upper inner thighs to facilitate a "connection" to the anterior pelvic floor and maintenance

of neutral hip alignment during the exercise. The ball is not to be squeezed, but merely held in place by the thighs sinking into the sides of the ball. Correct for neutral spine position, then cue a recruitment of the lumbopelvic and segmental thoracic stabilizers. Ask the patient to gently fold at the lower sternum and roll slightly back on the pelvis. Only a small movement is required. The patient is then asked to slowly rotate the thorax to the right and left, imagining that the rib cage is a lid on a jar that is turning while the jar (pelvis) stays still. The therapist provides manual feedback to ensure that the distance between the rib cage and iliac crests does not change and that no lateral shift or collapse of the thorax occurs during the rotation.

2) Bridge and Rotate (see Video Clip 7.32): The patient starts in crook lying. Check for lateral costal expansion during breathing. At the end of a breath out, cue the lumbopelvic stabilizers and the thoracic stabilizers, then instruct the patient to roll the pelvis back into a posterior pelvic tilt by pushing through the feet and lifting the hips off the floor. Cue a continued lumbar spine flexion as the hips are lifted. The midthorax remains on the floor. At the top of the "bridge" position, the patient is asked to release the hips and pelvis into a neutral pelvic tilt position ("let the buttocks drop and the hip creases fold"), creating a neutral lumbar lordosis. Once this is mastered, pelvic rotation under the thorax is added ("rotate the jar under the lid"). Cue a folding of the hip as the pelvis is slowly rotated to one side; to return to neutral, have the patient think of drawing the pelvis up from just inside the ASIS. Repeat the rotation to the opposite side. Movement must be controlled through both phases of the rotation. Return to the starting position by flexing the thorax ("let the chest go heavy"), then flexing the lumbar spine ("bring your low back down to the bed"), and finally releasing into a neutral lumbar lordosis ("let the pelvis tilt forward and the buttocks go wide"). A ball between the upper inner thighs can be used to facilitate control during the exercise.

Integrated functional kinetic chain

1) Low to High Pulleys (see Video Clip 7.33): This exercise integrates congruent rotation through multiple joints in a functional kinetic chain. The movement can be performed from low to high (flexion to extension) or from high to low (extension to flexion). The feet need to be able to pivot to allow movement through the whole chain; start with the feet facing the pulleys and then finish the movement with the feet pointing 180° from the start position. Aim to maintain the normal sagittal curves of the spine throughout (flexion and extension should occur at the hips and knees). The arms start low at the pulleys by flexing at the hips and knees, then rotation occurs through the legs, pelvis, and thorax as the arms are taken in a diagonal extension and elevation pattern, the front hip and knee extends and weight is transferred to the other leg. There should be no segmental shifting or anteroposterior loss of curves in the spine. The goal is a smooth controlled transition and integration of the rotation and extension at all joints along the chain. Use only light resistance as the focus is on control.

The final progression is the simulation of work and sport-specific maneuvers that require integration of movement through several joints. As mentioned previously, component parts of these complex maneuvers can be used as exercises in earlier stages in the stabilization program, when they are appropriate. Now is the time to practice the complete maneuver, but modified for speed and load. Start with low speed and low loads until control of the integrated movement is achieved, then progress to the speeds and loads that the functional task requires. Continue to concurrently practice low load and low speed tasks to ensure segmental and multisegmental control with the local stabilizing system. The ability to consciously isolate the segmental muscle contraction at the dysfunctional thoracic levels should be regularly checked and monitored throughout the progressions through the rehabilitation program, as episodes of recurrent pain and changed motor patterns can affect this ability to "connect" to the local system.

REFERENCES

Andriacchi T, Schultz A, Belytschko T, Galante J 1974 A model for studies of mechanical interactions between the human spine and rib cage. J. Biomechanics 7:497

Arendt-Nielsen L, Graven-Nielsen T, Svarrer H, Svensson P 1996 The influence of low back pain on muscle activity and coordination during gait: a clinical and experimental study. Pain. 64(2):231

Ashton-Miller J A, Howard D, DeLancey J O L 2001 The functional anatomy of the female pelvic floor and stress continence control system. Scand J. Urol Nephrol Suppl 207

Barker P J, Briggs C A 1999 Attachments of the posterior layer of the lumbar fascia. Spine 24:1757

Ben-Haim SA, Saidel GM: Mathematical model of chest wall mechanics: A phenomenological approach. Annals of Biomedical Engineering 1990; 18:37.

Bergmark A 1989 Stability of the lumbar spine. A study in mechanical engineering. Acta Orthopedica Scandinavia 230 (60):20

Bo K, Stein R 1994 Needle EMG registration of striated urethral wall and pelvic floor muscle activity patterns during cough, valsalva, abdominal, hip adductor, and gluteal muscles contractions in nulliparous healthy females. Neurourology and Urodynamics 13:35

Bogduk N 1997 Clinical anatomy of the lumbar spine and sacrum, 3rd edn. Churchill Livingstone, New York

Brown C W, Deffer P A, Akmakjian J, Donaldson D H, Brugman J L 1992 The natural history of thoracic disc herniation. Spine 17:6 Supplement

Bullock-Saxton J E, Janda V, Bullock M I 1994 The influence of ankle sprain injury on muscle activation during hip extension. Int J Sports Med. 15(6)330

Bump R C, Hurt G W, Fantl J A, Wyman J F 1991 Assessment of Kegel pelvic muscle exercise performance after brief verbal instruction. Am J Obstet Gynecol 165:322

Butler D S 2000 The sensitive nervous system. NOI group Publications, Adelaide, Australia

Buyruk H M, Snijders C J, Vleeming A, Laméris J S, Holland W P J, Stam H J 1995b The measurements of sacroiliac joint stiffness with colour doppler imaging: a study on healthy subjects. European Journal of Radiology 21:117

Buyruk H M, Stam H J, Snijders C J, Lameris J S, Holland W P Stijnen W P 1999 Measurement of sacroiliac joint stiffness in peripartum pelvic pain patients with Doppler imaging of vibrations (DIV). Eur J Obstet Gynecol Reprod Biol 83(2):159

Buyruk H M, Stam H J, Snijders C J, Vleeming A, Lameris J S, Holland W P J 1997 Measurement of sacroiliac joint stiffness with color Doppler imaging and the importance of asymmetric stiffness in sacroiliac pathology. In: Vleeming A, Mooney V, Dorman T, Snijders C, Stoeckart R (eds) Movement, stability and low back pain. Churchill Livingstone, Edinburgh, ch 24, p297

Buyruk H M, Stam H J, Snijders C J, Vleeming A, Laméris J S, Holland W P J 1995a The use of colour doppler imaging for the assessment of sacroiliac joint stiffness: a study on embalmed human pelvises. European Journal of Radiology 21:112

Carmichael J P 1987 Inter and intra examiner reliability of palpation for sacroiliac joint dysfunction. Journal Manipulative Physical Therapy 10(4):164

Carriere B 1996 Therapeutic exercise and self-correction programs. In: The thoracic spine and rib cage. Ed. Flynn T W Butterworth-Heinemann

Comerford M J, Mottram S L 2001 Movement and stability dysfunction – contemporary developments. Manual Therapy 6(1):15

Constantinou C E, Govan D E 1982 Spatial distribution and timing of transmitted and reflexly generated urethral pressures in healthy women. Journal of Urology 127:964

Danneels L A, Vanderstraeten G, Cambier D, Witvrouw E, Raes H, de Cuyper H 2001 A randomized clinical trial of three rehabilitation programs for the lumbar multifidus in patients with chronic low back pain. In: Proceedings from the 4th Interdisciplinary World Congress on Low Back & Pelvic Pain. Montreal, Canada p219

Dangaria T, Naesh O 1998 Changes in cross-sectional area of psoas major muscle in unilateral sciatic caused by disc herniation. Spine 23(8)928

Danneels LA, Vanderstraeten GG, Cambier DC, Witvrouw EE, De Cuyper HJ 2000 CT Imaging of Trunk Muscles in Chronic Low Back Pain Patients and Healthy Control Subjects. European Spine 9(4):266

Davis P R 1959 The medial inclination of the human thoracic intervertebral articular facets. Journal of Anatomy 93:68

DeRosa C 2001 Functional anatomy of the lumbar spine and sacroiliac joint. In: Proceedings from the 4th Interdisciplinary World Congress on Low Back & Pelvic Pain. Montreal, Canada p3

DeTroyer A D 1989 The mechanism of the inspiratory expansion of the rib cage. J Lab Clin Med 114(2):97

Donisch E W, Basmajian J V 1972 Electromyography of deep back muscles in man. Am J Anat 133(1):25

Dreyfuss P, Dreyer S, Griffin J, Hoffman J, Walsh N 1994 Positive sacroiliac screening tests in asymptomatic adults. Spine 19:1138

Dreyfuss P, Michaelsen M, Pauza D, McLarty J, Bogduk N 1996 The value of history and physical examination in diagnosing sacroiliac joint pain. Spine 21:2594

Farrell J, Drye C, Koury M 1994 Therapeutic exercise for back pain. In Twomey LT & Taylor JR (Eds.): Physical therapy of the low back, 2nd edn. low back. Eds. Twomey L T, Taylor J R, Churchill Livingstone, New York p 379

Gibbons S 2002 Rehabilitation of the stability function of psoas major. In: Orthopaedic Division Review. CPA publication January/February p9

Giles L G F & Singer K P 2000 Clinical anatomy and management of thoracic spine pain. Butterworth Heinemann, Oxford

Gracovetsky S 1990 Musculoskeletal function of the spine. In: Multiple muscle systems: Biomechanics and Movement Organization. Winters JM, Woo SLY

(eds) Springer Verlag, New York

Gunn C C 1999 The Gunn approach to the treatment of chronic pain. Intramuscular stimulation for myofasical pain of radiculopathic origin. Churchill Livingstone, London

Hall C M, Brody L T 1999 Therapeutic exercise moving toward function. Philadelphia: Lippincott Williams & Wilkins.

Hayashi K, Yabuki T 1985 Origin of the uncus of Luschka's joint in the cervical spine. JBJS 67A:788

Herzog W, Read L, Conway P J W, Shaw L D, McEwen M C 1989 Reliability of motion palpation procedures to detect sacroiliac joint fixations. Journal Manipulative Physical Therapy 12(2):86

Hides J A, Stokes M J, Saide M, Jull G A, Cooper D H 1994 Evidence of lumbar multifidus muscles wasting ipsilateral to symptoms in patients with acute/subacute low back pain. Spine 19(2):165

Hides J A, Richardson C A, Jull G A 1996 Multifidus recovery is not automatic following resolution of acute first episode low back pain. Spine 21(23):2763

Hides J A, Jull G A, Richardson C A 2001 Long-term effects of specific stabilizing exercises for first-episode low back pain. Spine 26(11):E243

Hodges P W, Richardson C A 1996 Inefficient muscular stabilization of the lumbar spine associated with low back pain. A motor control evaluation of transversus abdominis. Spine 21(22):2640

Hodges P W, Richardson C A 1997a Contraction of the abdominal muscles associated with movement of the lower limb. Physical Therapy 77:132

Hodges P W 1997b Feedforward contraction of transversus abdominis is not influenced by the direction of arm movement. Experimental Brain Research, 114:362

Hodges P W, Gandevia S C 2000 Changes in intra-abdominal pressure during postural and respiratory activation of the human diaphragm. Journal Applied Physiology 89:967

Holstege G, Bandler R, Saper C B 1996 The emotional motor system. Elsevier Science

Janda V 1978 Muscles, central nervous motor regulation and back problems. In: The neurobiologic mechanisms in manipulative therapy. Ed. I M Korr. Plenum Press, New York

Jull G A, Richardson C A 2000 Motor control problems in patients with spinal pain: A new direction for therapeutic exercise. Journal of Manipulative and Physiological Therapeutics. 23(2):115

Kaigle A M, Wessberg P, Hansson T H 1998 Muscular and kinematic behavior of the lumbar spine during flexion-extension. J Spinal Disord. 11(2):163

Laslett M, Williams W 1994 The reliability of selected pain provocation tests for sacroiliac joint pathology. Spine 19(11):1243

Lee D G 1993 Biomechanics of the thorax: a clinical model of in vivo function. Journal of Manual and Manipulative Therapy 1:13

Lee D G 1994 Biomechanics of the thorax. Chapter 3 in: Physical Therapy of the Cervical and Thoracic Spine. Ed: Ruth Grant. Churchill Livingstone, New York

Lee D G 1999 The Pelvic Girdle, 2nd edition. Churchill Livingstone. Edinburgh

Lee D G 2001 Imagery for Core Stabilization – an educational video. DGL Physiotherapist Corp., www.dianelee.ca

Lee D G, Vleeming A 1998 Impaired load transfer through the pelvic girdle – a new model of altered neutral zone function. In: 3rd Interdisciplinary World Congress on Low Back and Pelvic Pain. November 19-21, Vienna, Austria. p76

Lee D G, Vleeming A 2002 Management of pelvic joint pain and dysfunction. In: 3rd edition of Modern Manual Therapy eds. Jull & Palastanga, Elsevier Science (at press)

Levin S M 1997 A different approach to the mechanics of the human pelvis: tensegrity. In A Vleeming, V Mooney, T Dorman, C Snijders, R Stoeckart (Eds.), Movement, Stability and Low Back Pain. Churchill Livingstone, London p 157

Lowcock J Thoracic Joint Stability and Clinical Stress Tests. Proceedings of the Canadian Orthopaedic Manipulative Physiotherapists, 1990, Orthopaedic Division of the Canadian Physiotherapy Association Newsletter November/December 1991 p15

MacConaill M A, Basmajian J V 1977 Muscles and movements; a basis for human kinesiology. 2nd edn. Kreiger, New York

Mattila M, Hurme M, Alaranta H, Paljarvi L, Kalimo H, Falck B, Lehto M, Einola S, Jarvinen M 1986 The multifidus muscle in patients with lumbar disc herniation. Spine 11(7):732

McArdle WD, Katch FI, Katch VL 1991. Exercise physiology. Energy, Nutrition, and Human Performance. 3rd edn. Lea & Febiger, Malvern PA

McGill S 2002 Low back disorders. Evidence-based prevention and rehabilitation. Human Kinetics. Champaign, Ilinois

Mens J M A, Vleeming A, Snijders C J, Koes B J, Stam H J 2001 Reliability and validity of the active straight leg raise test in posterior pelvic pain since pregnancy. Spine 26(10):1167

Mens J M A, Vleeming A, Snijders C J, Stam H J 1997 Active straight leg raising test: a clinical approach to the load transfer function of the pelvic girdle. In: Vleeming A, Mooney V, Dorman T, Snijders C, Stoeckart R (eds) Movement, stability and low back pain. Churchill Livingstone, Edinburgh

Mens J M A, Vleeming A, Snijders C J, Stam H J, Ginai A Z 1999 The active straight leg raising test and mobility of the pelvic joints. European Spine 8:468

Meyers T W 2001 Anatomy Trains. Churchill Livingstone, Edinburgh

Morris J M, Benner G, Lucas D B 1962 An electromyographic study of the intrinsic muscles of the back in man. J Anat Lond 96(4):509

Moseley G L, Hodges P W, Gandevia S C. 2002 Deep and superficial fibers of the lumbar multifidus muscle are differentially active during voluntary arm movements. Spine 27(2):E29

Murphy M 1992 The future of the body: explorations into the further evolution of human nature. Tarcher Putnam, New York

O'Sullivan P, Twomey L, Allison G 1997. Evaluation of specific stabilising exercise in the treatment of chronic low back pain with radiological diagnosis of spondylolysis and spondylolisthesis. Spine 15(24):2959

O'Sullivan P 2000 Lumbar segmental instability – diagnosis and specific exercise management. In: Proceedings of the 7th Scientific Conference of IFOMT. Perth, Australia

Panjabi M M 1992 The stabilizing system of the spine. I: Function, dysfunction, adaptation, and enhancement. Part II. Neutral zone and instability hypothesis. Journal of Spinal Disorders 5(4):383

Panjabi M M, Brand R A, White A A 1976 Mechanical properties of the human thoracic spine. JBJS 58A:642

Panjabi M M, Hausfeld J N, White A A 1981 A biomechanical study of the ligamentous stability of the thoracic spine in man. Acta orthop. scan. 52:315

Penning L, Wilmink J T 1987 Rotation of the cervical spine – A CT study in normal subjects. Spine 12:732

Primal 3D Interactive Series 2000, Primal Pictures, www.anatomy.tv, London

Radebold A, Cholewicki J, Panjabi M M, Patel T C 2000 Muscle response pattern to sudden trunk loading in healthy individuals and in patients with chronic low back pain. Spine 25(8):947

Richardson C A, Jull G A, Hodges P W, Hides J A 1999 Therapeutic exercise for spinal segmental stabilization in low back pain – scientific basis and clinical approach. Churchill Livingstone, Edinburgh

Richardson C A, Snijders C J, Hides J A, Damen L, Pas M S, Storm J 2002 The relationship between the transversely oriented abdominal muscles, sacroiliac joint mechanics and low back pain. Spine 27(4):399-405

Rizk N N 1980 A new description of the anterior abdominal wall in man and mammals. Journal Anatomy 131:373

Sahrmann S 2001 Diagnosis and Treatment of Movement Impairment Syndromes, Elsevier Science

Sapolsky R M, Alberts R C, Altmann J 1997a Hypercortisolism associated with social subordinance isolation among wild baboons. Archives General Psychiatry 54(12):1137

Sapolsky R M, Spencer E M 1997b Insulin growth factor 1 is suppressed in socially subordinate male baboons. American Journal Physiology 273 (4 Pt 2):1346

Saumarez R C 1986 An analysis of possible movements of human upper rib cage. Journal of Applied Physiology 60:678

Sapsford R R, Hodges P W, Richardson C A, Cooper D H, Markwell S J, Jull G A 2001 Co-activation of the abdominal and pelvic floor muscles during voluntary exercises. Neurourology and Urodynamics 20:31

Saumarez R C 1986 An analysis of possible movements of human upper rib cage. Journal of Applied Physiology 60:678

Singer K P, Goh S 2000 Anatomy of the thoracic spine. In: Clinical anatomy and management of thoracic spine pain. Eds. Giles L F G, Singer K P. Butterworth-Heinemann, Oxford

Snijders C J, Vleeming A, Stoeckart R 1993 Transfer of lumbosacral load to iliac bones and legs Part 1: Biomechanics of self-bracing of the sacroiliac joints and its significance for treatment and exercise. Part 2: Loading of the sacroiliac joints when lifting in a stooped posture. Clinical Biomechanics 8: 285

Sternberg E M 2000 The balance within. The science connecting health and emotions. W. H. Freeman and Co, New York

Uhlig Y, Weber B R, Grob D, Muntener M 1995 Fiber composition and fiber transformations in neck muscles of patients with dysfunction of the cervical spine. Journal of Orthopaedic Research 13:240

Urquhart D, Hodges P, Story I 2001 Regional variation in transversus abdominis recruitment. In: 4th Interdisciplinary World Congress on Low Back and Pelvic Pain Proceedings. Montreal, Canada p358

Vleeming A, Stoeckart R, Volkers A C W, Snijders C J 1990a Relation between form and function in the sacroiliac joint. 1: Clinical anatomical aspects. Spine 15(2):130

Vleeming A, Volkers A C W, Snijders C J, Stoeckart R 1990b Relation between form and function in the sacroiliac joint. 11: Biomechanical aspects. Spine 15(2):133

Vleeming A, Pool-Goudzwaard A L, Stoeckart R, Wingerden J P van, Snijders C J 1995a The posterior layer of the thoracolumbar fascia: its function in load transfer from spine to legs. Spine 20:753

Vleeming A, Snijders C J, Stoeckart R, Mens J M A 1995b A new light on low back pain. In: Proceedings from the 2nd Interdisciplinary World Congress on Low Back Pain. San Diego

Willems JM, Jull GA, Ng JKF 1996 An in vivo study of the primary and coupled rotations of the thoracic spine. Clinical Biomechanics 2(6): 311

Williams P, Warwick R, Dyson M, Bannister L H 1989 Grays anatomy. 37th edn. Churchill Livingstone, Edinburgh

Wingerden J P van , Vleeming A, Buyruk H M, Raissadat K 2001 Muscular contribution to force closure ; sacroiliac joint stabilization in vivo. In: Proceedings from the 4th Interdisciplinary World Congress on Low Back & Pelvic Pain. Montreal, Canada p153

Yue G, Cole K J 1992 Strength increase from the motor programme: Comparison of training with maximal voluntary and imagined muscle contractions. Journal of Neurophysiology 67(5): 1114-1123

Instructions for viewing the video clips on this CD-ROM:

1. To maximize the viewing of the video clips, change your display setting in your computer to a screen resolution of 800 X 600 as follows:

   a. Select START

   b. CONTROL PANEL

   c. DISPLAY

   d. SETTINGS

   e. Choose a SCREEN RESOLUTION of 800 X 600

   f. APPLY

2. Place the CDROM in your CDROM drive, it should automatically start up. If it doesn't, go to MY COMPUTER from your START menu, select your CDROM drive and click on autorun.exe.

3. To play the desired video clip, click on the chapter button, then select the category and click on the specific clip from the pull down menus.

4. To change the screen size of the video, click on the SCREEN SIZE button. To minimize the screen size, click on the SCREEN SIZE button again.

5. Select EXIT to quit.

NOTE: THERE IS NO AUDIO ASSOCIATED WITH THESE VIDEO CLIPS.